GONE

GONE

A Memoir of Love, Body,
and Taking Back My Life

Linda K. Olson

SHE WRITES PRESS

Published 2020
Printed in the United States of America
ISBN: 978-1-63152-789-0
ISBN: 978-1-63152-790-6
Library of Congress Control Number: 2020907892

For information, address:
She Writes Press
1569 Solano Ave #546
Berkeley, CA 94707

Interior design by Tabitha Lahr

She Writes Press is a division of SparkPoint Studio, LLC.

Dedicated to:

Dave—for making me feel like a woman, allowing me to become independent again, and loving me unconditionally.

Tiffany and Brian—without you, my life would have been incomplete.

Contents

PROLOGUE:

A Daughter's Perspective

....

I thumbed the worn edges of the envelope Adrian had given me. For three weeks, I'd refrained from examining its contents, knowing that I would need some time alone to process what I would see. Adrian, a dear friend of my grandparents, and I had hoped to get a chance to sit down and record her memories of the past thirty years but had not been able to find time. Instead, she'd offered to dig up some photographs for me, promising a detailed discussion in the near future.

I slid my thumb under the flap and pulled out a thick card. Inside it were eight photographs and a note written in Adrian's impeccable cursive. It read:

> *Dear Tiffany,*
> *Here are the photos I promised you. The one of your*
> *mom taken the evening before the trip is not good,*
> *but it is a treasure. We were all having drinks in our*

house. All of our lives changed the next day. It has been a privilege to be part of your family and this incredible journey.

Love,
Adrian

I have always loved looking at photographs taken of my parents and grandparents when I was a baby, toddler, and adolescent, not to see how I've grown, but to see the transformation in these people who have always been old to me. It is jarring that they were young once.

I picked up the stack of pictures and examined the first one, taken on Sunday, August 26, 1979. In it, my mother is twenty-nine years old, three months shy of her thirtieth birthday. Ten months younger than I was sitting there that day.

Adrian was right: the photograph is rather poor quality. It was taken haphazardly, as though the photographer were unaware of the moment he was memorializing, which he was—they all were. There are three people in the frame. My mother sits on the floor in front of an empty fireplace, facing the photographer. She is slender, dressed in a dark blue, long-sleeved shirt and white pants, her legs tucked under her, right hand resting in her lap. My Uncle Mark sits to her right, dressed in jeans and a yellow T-shirt, staring absently at the brown shag carpeting covering the floor. The third person sits with her back to the photographer, legs outstretched, gin and tonic in hand.

The photograph was taken in Stuttgart, Germany, in the apartment that Adrian and her husband, Johnny, occupied at the US Army garrison. My grandparents were stationed there as well. The subjects of the photograph, those whose faces were captured, appear tired and have probably just finished one of my grandmother's famous gourmet meals. Travel guides spread in front of them, they are finalizing the details of their trip to Berchtesgaden, planned for the following day.

As my father tells it, the morning of the trip was overcast, with occasional light rain—typical Central European summer weather. My parents, grandparents, and uncle, with his then wife, piled into a Volkswagen van for a leisurely drive through southern Bavaria. Stopping in Ulm for lunch, my father, my mother, and my uncle made the dizzying climb to the top of the tallest steeple in Europe. My mother—strong, lithe, and athletic—had no problem keeping up with her husband and his brother, both marathon runners. My father recalls that this was the last time his wife of almost two years would use her lovely, slender legs.

Continuing on their journey after a few wrong turns, they found themselves on a steep, winding road, trying to find their way back on course. The road flattened to cross the railroad tracks, and my grandfather downshifted. The van stalled. The men piled out the front door facing away from the oncoming train. The women failed to open the side door in the back seat, but my mother scrambled into the front and fell out onto the tracks. My father automatically turned midstride to go back to help her, certain they were going to die. Straddling the tracks, he managed to grab her under her arms. As he turned away with her in his arms, the train made impact with the van. He felt his arms pulled downward as my mother was crushed underneath the van. He was tossed aside, unconscious.

My mother lost both legs, amputated a few inches above the knees, and her right arm, amputated at the shoulder. This is how I have always known her. I spent the first few years of my life thinking that was how mothers were supposed to be. I felt sorry for the children who didn't have a nightly wheelchair ride or butt-walk races on the weekend. They missed playing with canes and prostheses and may never have known how far a wheelchair can slide on an icy sidewalk.

As I got older, her disability became a source of a sort of pride for me. I hated other people staring at her as she rolled by in her wheelchair or marched along with her awkward tin-soldier gait, their heads on a swivel as she passed. I wanted everyone to know that her disability was only physical, not mental, and that she could do everything that everyone else could do. I would stare just as hard right back at them until they turned away uncomfortably.

I was and still am possessive of her. As a child, I could not wait until I was strong enough to carry her and put her legs on. My father would patiently stand by as I tugged and pulled fruitlessly on my mother's stockings, trying to yank them off her legs and out through the hole of her prostheses. The day I was able to get her legs on was as exciting as my first trip to Disneyland. My father made lifting her eighty-pound, legless body look like picking up a sack of feathers. It wasn't. I tried and tried until I could finally, at about age fourteen, carry her down to the beach. Next came carrying her with her legs on, usually up and down stairs. Her legs added about twenty pounds but gave me something to hold on to. "No, thanks. I don't need any help" became my mantra when going places with her. I became a pack mule of sorts and relished the role. I felt needed and important, able to help my mother go places and do things that would have been much more difficult, if not impossible, for her to do on her own.

Looking at the photograph from an adult's perspective, I was humbled by this young woman whose life was destroyed and re-created in a matter of seconds. I wondered if I would be able to pull off such a resurrection with as much élan as she did and still does.

That was the first photograph I'd seen of my mother as an adult before the accident. I do not know the person with legs in it. That image and my current image of my mother are incongruous. I was frustrated that the photograph was so subdued and still. I wished that it showed her midrun, midjump, or midkick, any demonstration of her boundless energy innervating her real legs. I wanted to poke at the photograph and force her to stand, to show me that those legs really did work.

The second photograph in the bunch shows my mother and father, both sitting in wheelchairs in the courtyard of the hospital in Salzburg. It shows the mother I recognize. She is wearing a lacy white camisole nightgown and is cocooned in billowing white sheets. Her sternum is supported by a cruciform brace, and the bruised and stitched stump of her right arm is exposed. The part of the photograph I recognize most is her grin. Holding the armrest of her wheelchair with her left arm, she sits straight up, laughing at someone or something in front of her. My mother's being serious is a rare sight for me and usually means trouble. Her high spirits clearly were not lost with her limbs. My father sits to her left, looking as though someone has just gotten hit by a train. No doubt he had already mentally rearranged his life and was regimenting the next few months of rehabilitation boot camp. This is typical. My father's seriousness almost balances my mother's ridiculousness. His intensity and drive, coupled with my mother's energy and positivity and their combined determination, are what got them through it all. My grandmother, smiling, leans with her arms around my father's neck, her right hand midpat on his shoulder. Adrian's long arms span all three of them. That photograph exemplifies the attitude that our family and those close to us have always adopted about the accident: "If you can do it, I can do it."

I thumbed through the rest of the photographs, which must have been taken a week or so after the accident. My mother's family had arrived, and everyone had begun the process of healing and trying to return to a semblance of normalcy. I sensed a heaviness in the subjects and not for the first time wondered how this incident truly affected them.

The last photo shows my father kissing my mother, a smile playing at her lips. It is a glimpse, early on in the struggle before them, of the happiness and strength they would share with everyone around them. It is my favorite.

CHAPTER 1:

The Day Our Life

Went Off the Rails

....

"We've gotta move," I screamed at the driver as I shook the back of the seat. "Get off the track, Jack. A train is coming!"

I saw the monster bearing down on us through the left-side windows of a borrowed VW van. The whistle's crescendo was deafening. *We're going to die. I'm only twenty-nine. I'm not ready to die.* In seconds, the men had clambered out of the front passenger-side door. I clawed at the metal sliding-door handle next to me and yanked it back. Nothing happened.

Dave, his brother, and their dad had been riding in the front seat. His mother, sister-in-law, and I were in the middle seat behind them. The sound of my pounding heart blocked all noise except the voice in my head. *Dave is out there somewhere.*

I grabbed the handle again and jerked hard. Nothing.

The front door. All I had to do was jump forward, slide out, stand up, and run. *I can make it!*

1

I catapulted over the front seat, landed awkwardly, and, before I could catch myself, tumbled out the open passenger door onto the tracks. The only thing standing between me and the train was the van, with my mother- and sister-in-law still inside. I scrambled frantically to right myself.

Suddenly, my chest felt tight and I was lifted off the tracks. I opened my eyes. Dave's face was inches from mine; his strong arms were wrapped around me. *He's going to save me!* I could hear again. Dave was gasping for breath. His arms tightened around me, and then he was gone.

In one earth-shaking, deafening instant, the locomotive smashed into the van, pushing me down onto my back across the track. The blue sky above me disappeared as the van folded over me, blocking the color and light as the train hit it. Time morphed. Seconds jumbled and tumbled. Time ran away and disappeared.

I took a deep breath and held it. *If I let it out, I might never breathe again. I must hold it . . . hold it . . . hold it. Till death do us part . . .*

The train pushed me down the tracks. I felt nothing.

When it stopped, I heard new sounds. Human voices. Indecipherable words. I didn't care what they were saying. If I could hear them, I was still alive.

The hands of time began to move again. Something was happening. I heard the scraping of metal on metal. The train was backing up. Someone shouted. People grunted and strained to lift the van. The terrible weight pressing down on me lessened. I found myself squinting against the late-afternoon sun.

I took a deep breath and felt a sharp pain in my chest. *Pain is good! Breathing is good. What are they saying?*

Then I remembered. I was in Germany. *German! They're speaking German! That's why I can't understand them. Maybe I don't have brain damage. They pulled the van off me. I'm alive!*

I smiled at the panicked-looking faces hovering over me. They did not reciprocate. Heads turned away. Hands held me down. My mind raced. *Am I paralyzed?* I was afraid to move. I didn't want to know. But I smiled. It's what I always did, and the only thing I could do for these horror-struck strangers. *I'm okay*, I tried to convey. *Don't worry; I'll be okay.*

No one was speaking English, so I had to work it out on my own: I was conscious, my glasses were still on my face, and I could see clearly. People swirled around me, some with purpose, others plodding mindlessly, as if through movement they could somehow make sense of the scene before them. I didn't feel part of it either; it was as if I were watching a movie.

The scream of a siren got closer and closer. I looked around, wondering if there were other people on the ground. *Who is the ambulance coming for?* There were six of us in the van. *Where is everyone?*

Out of the corner of my eye, I saw a shoe, then, farther away, another. One was Dave's. *Where is Dave?* The other was light tan with a rubber sole. It looked an awful lot like the new ones I'd bought for the trip.

An ambulance stopped abruptly very near where I lay against the hot tracks. Its doors flew open, and medical personnel rushed over. They tied tourniquets around my right shoulder and high up on my legs. I heard the whooshing air of a blood pressure cuff as it tightened around my left arm.

I stared at each face. They looked at each other and shook their heads. "My blood pressure is always low," I said. *Why do they look so worried?*

I knew from my medical training that if blood pressure got too low, the team responsible for saving my life might start to lose hope and motivation. I smiled and repeated, more slowly and more loudly, "My . . . blood . . . pressure . . . is . . . always . . . low! It's okay!"

Big men gingerly slipped their arms under me and transferred me to a stretcher. An attendant picked up my still neatly tied shoe and walked toward me. He placed it at the end of my gurney. Conveniently, my foot was still inside it. Someone else put part of a leg next to it. The knot in my stomach twisted tighter.

I tried to sit up but couldn't. I pushed again. Nothing happened. *Why can't I raise my arm?* The right sleeve of my dark green velour shirt looked fine, not so much as a tear. My right hand, attached to my arm, lay motionless beside me on the gurney. My arm looked perfect as it protruded from the sleeve cuff. It was, however, hanging loose inside, unattached to my body.

I closed my eyes.

The ambulance swayed as it sped around mountain curves. The paramedics rocked back and forth in time with the motion of the vehicle, silent as they steadied my gurney. Time seemed to fly away again until we slowed and stopped. The ambulance doors were yanked open, and the low-hanging sun temporarily blinded me. A man in a US military uniform poked his head in toward me. "I'm Dr. . . ." His eyes quickly scanned the scene in front of him. "Let's get her out!"

He's speaking English! He leaned over, pulled the sheet off me, and pressed his fingers against my neck, feeling for a carotid pulse while he looked at the bloody tourniquets tied on three of my extremities.

"How are you?" he asked curtly.

Not wanting to state the obvious, I flashed a smile and said, "Fine."

The doctor in me assessed my situation: foot in shoe, leg on gurney, loose arm in sleeve. *I'm going to die. I'm going to bleed to death.* In some ways, I was fine—fine with dying. I wasn't sure I wanted to live like that.

There was a brief silence as the doctor stepped away from the door, then an exchange of words that floated over my head. He pulled the sheet back over me as he said, "We can't keep you here. You need to get to surgery as fast as possible. We're calling ahead to the trauma hospital in Salzburg and alerting them to prepare for your arrival." He looked deep into my eyes and squeezed my remaining hand tightly. "Hurry and good luck! We'll be praying for you."

I watched the doors slam shut. I did want to live. *Maybe they'll get me to Salzburg in time. Surely they wouldn't have sent us off if there wasn't any hope.* I looked at the faces of the men in the ambulance. *If they have hope, I have hope. I'll fool them as long as I can.*

"I'll be okay. My blood pressure is fine. It's always low," I reminded them. *Don't give up on me, guys. Please don't give up on me.*

It was a twenty-minute race to the trauma hospital across the passport-controlled border between Germany and Austria. The rapid, deep, up-down, two-note sound of the siren provided the soundtrack for the scene as the ambulance sped me toward my date with a room full of surgeons. *I'm going to die; I'm going to live. I'm going to die; I'm going to live. I'm going to die; I'm going to live.*

We stopped abruptly, and the doors clanged open. Out and down I went on the gurney, gripping it with the only extremity I had left. I fought to open my eyes, but they were too heavy. Everything was spinning. The sharp smell of alcohol and clipped, ordered speech of people told me I must be in an emergency room. Time was running out.

I was fading as I felt the sting of a needle in the skin under my clavicle, and the ER doctor put a catheter into my subclavian vein. As a physician, I knew this meant serious trouble. Then there was nothing.

~

Slowly, I became aware of the soft beeping of a cardiac monitor, speaking the universal language of medicine. I pulled against the weight of my eyelids, willing them to move. When they finally opened a crack, the glare hurt. I winced, closed them again, and listened. Subdued voices floated over me while squeaks from rubber-soled shoes moved quickly around the room. The beeping had a steady, reassuring beat. The voices, on the other hand, were unintelligible, so I made a bigger effort to open my eyes. Across the room, a clock on the wall said it was four. *Probably in the morning.* It was pitch black outside the window.

Concentrating with all my might, I heard and saw everything that had happened. *Was that yesterday: the van stopping, a train, Dave picking me up, the loudest noise I've ever heard, an ambulance, my foot, part of a leg, and an arm disconnected from my body?*

I took several deep breaths, opened my eyes, and forced myself to look down. A tent-like apparatus covered the lower half of me. I allowed my eyes to scan the contours of my body. My left arm lay at my side on top of the sheet. Under the sheet covering me, I could make out the familiar curve of my waist and flat stomach, but just below my hips, the fabric made an abrupt plunge to meet the mattress. It was true. Both my legs were gone. My right arm was gone. Life as I knew it was gone.

Images of Dave's face floated all around me. I clenched my fist and tried to make them go away but drifted back to the beginning.

~

I'd noticed him the first day of medical school, the blond, handsome guy with the cute mustache and sideburns who sat below me in the anatomy amphitheater. He was in the front row of every class, taking extensive notes, staring intently at the slides or blackboard, and watching the professor. He was so focused that he didn't notice my considerable efforts at flirting.

He grew up relying on sports to serve as an emotional outlet and to help him to maintain an even keel in life. But medical school was so time-consuming that he needed exercise he could do at odd hours and that didn't require money or other people's participation.

So, running became his thing. Starting at 5:00 a.m., before the Inland Empire heat and smog settled in, he ran in the dark on silent, isolated roads through orange grove after orange grove. If you'd passed him on the road, you would have seen him talking to himself, his arms pumping and hands gesticulating, his mind racing ahead of his feet.

If you'd asked him why he was running, he would have said that it calmed him and helped temper his impulsivity for the rest of the day. This was the 1970s. Researchers were just discovering the opioid neuropeptides (now known as endorphins) that eventually inspired the term "runner's high." Dave is living proof that it is an effective process. When he doesn't run, he is hard to live with. When he runs, he is easy to love.

By the end of med school, he averaged thirty-five miles per week. I rode my mint-green Bianchi racing bike alongside him whenever I could. We didn't talk. The effort the terrain required didn't allow it. Footfall by footfall, pedal stroke by pedal stroke, breath by breath, we were together yet separate. We'd become a team.

~

Daylight streamed in through the window. It was Tuesday, August 28—in medical jargon, post-op day one. In my mind, it was the first day of a different life. I'd been mentally preparing for it over the past few hours. I knew where I was. I knew what had happened. What I didn't know was how Dave was doing. I hadn't seen him since the accident, but I'd been told that he'd broken his ankle and been knocked out but would be okay.

Will he really? Will he be okay with having a severely disabled wife? He married a cute, slim doctor with whom he hiked, biked, and traveled. What if I can't do things with him anymore? What if I can't work? Why would he want to stick around?

In good times, Dave struggles with anger issues. I wondered what he would do when he saw the mangled, tiny version of Linda, the visible remains being only the face he'd loved to kiss and one arm—half of what I used to hug him with, half of what I used to play the organ and piano for him with, half the person he used to cook Julia Child recipes with. *Will he take out his anger on himself, or someone else . . . or me?*

I knew I was in stable condition because a nurse was carefully sponging my face with a warm, wet cloth, avoiding the scabs and scrapes, while another gently worked a comb through the tangles of my hair. How would my husband of only two years react to seeing me wrapped in bandages and missing my legs and right arm? I was grateful that the nurses were doing their best to make me presentable. I pulled my shoulders down, trying to make them look as level as possible, and sat up as straight as my bed and back brace would allow. *At least I look sort of normal from the shoulders up.*

The double doors swung open. I held my breath as Dave, gripping his crutches, hobbled in with his left leg in a walking cast. His blond hair was unruly. A brown hospital robe was cinched around his waist. Eyes fixed on me, he limped past the nurses' station and headed straight toward my cot, the only one occupying the long, seven-patient, old-school intensive care unit. He looked frail. The heat rose in my face. My chest tightened. I clenched my jaw and twisted the sheet in my fist, trying not to cry as I looked at his pale, haggard, unshaven face. *What is he thinking?*

I needed to be strong for him. I grinned as he crutched to my bedside while I silently rehearsed the two sentences I'd carefully crafted and memorized.

When he reached me, he slipped one of his hands under mine and with his other stroked the back of my hand. The gentleness of his touch on my wrist, across my knuckles, and down to my fingertips sent a familiar, warm sensation up my arm and across my chest. He gingerly bent over me, kissed my forehead, and pressed his cheek against mine. I could feel and hear his heartbeat and breath. As he straightened, I avoided his gaze, focusing instead on the empty space beyond the stumps of my thighs.

"I've been thinking about things," I began. "I'll understand if you don't want to stick around."

He shifted and let the crutches fall away from his body. I dared to look up and into his green eyes. Tears ran down his cheeks as he squeezed my hand. "Olsie, Olsie, Olsie, I didn't marry your arms and your legs. . . ." His voice cracked. "If you can do it, I can do it."

We were awash in a flood of emotions for several minutes. When the tide ebbed, Dave asked, "Do you know what happened to you?"

"I never lost consciousness," I replied. "I remember everything. I know I've lost both my legs and my arm."

I faltered and then forced myself to continue. "Wh. . . what happened to everyone else?"

His grip on my hand tightened. "You aren't going to believe this. . . you and I are the only ones that got hurt. When the train hit us, my mom and Carol were thrown into the back of the van and nothing happened to them. Mark and I and my dad got out safely before the impact."

He drew in a long breath, and I watched as the emotion cleared, making way for Dave the medical professional.

"Linda, is it okay if I do a neuro exam to see whether you have a spinal cord injury?"

"Yes, Dr. Dave," I said, winking away a remaining tear.

He slipped his hands under the protective bridge and stopped briefly to admire the precision with which the staff had wrapped and taped the surgical dressings that covered the ends of my thighs. "They did a wonderful job," he said, more to himself than to me. "Okay, Linda, can you feel this?" he asked as he gently touched the tops, sides, and bottoms of my left thigh.

"Yes, I can feel it," I said, happy to be feeling anything that a normal spinal cord would allow me to feel.

"What do you feel?"

"It feels like your finger is just barely touching my skin."

"I'm going to test for pain and lightly pinch you."

I felt a gentle pinch and nodded my head, relieved to have the information.

"Can you move your thighs comfortably?"

"Just a little," I said as I moved each one up and down and side to side.

"Do you feel any tingling or burning up here?" Dave asked as he softly drummed his fingers on my thighs.

"No, but I can still feel my lower legs and feet, and that's a tingling feeling," I said.

"I think you're good. No deficit that I can detect."

Satisfied that there wasn't any neurological damage, Dave stepped back into husband mode, pulling the sheet up over me and once again taking my hand in his.

We talked. We didn't talk about piano playing, the pipe organ, bicycling, hiking, skiing, or climbing the steps of the bell tower of the Ulm Cathedral, which we'd done the day before. We didn't talk about how I had often climbed barefoot up onto

Dave's shoes to reach up and give him a kiss. We talked about getting through the next few days and weeks. We focused on the new and the now: this afternoon, tomorrow.

"*Fünf Minuten*," announced a nurse from the station across the room. Technically, I was stable but still in critical condition. It had been less than twenty-four hours since the accident. The nurses wanted me to rest.

"If you can do it, I can do it," Dave said as he picked up his crutches and limped reluctantly to the double doors. He turned awkwardly to look at me one more time before stepping out into the bright hallway beyond the comfort of me and my bedside. I was pretty sure he was crying. I was.

"I love you," I murmured. And then I was alone, a tiny figure swaddled in white.

White sheets covered me. White pillows propped me up. Rolls and rolls of white gauze covered by white tape protected the ends of my severed arm and legs. Even my feelings were vanilla, kept at bay by powerful painkillers that let me float above all the whiteness. Nurses glided around me, whispering terse observations and orders in German. A central venous line, an IV, and a urinary catheter took care of most of my bodily functions.

All I had to do was rest. All I could do was think.

For the rest of the day, in a haze, I alternated between two personae: Dr. Olson and Linda. Looking around, I assessed my situation.

Legs:
- gone but somehow still here
- absence of legs from midthigh down—not okay

That was going to be a big problem. That would require a wheelchair. I was not okay with that. *People in wheelchairs are nobodies. There's no way I can spend the rest of my life in a wheelchair.*

Arm:

- have one left; nondominant
- doesn't hurt
- has full range of motion
- no scrapes or bruises
- all five fingers intact

It would take some practice and creativity, but I was sure I'd have a perfectly usable arm.

Back:

- hurts

Actually, it hurt like hell!

I'd asked to see the X-rays of my spine. The findings were obvious when I held them up to the light and looked at the lateral view. Instead of the normal, rectangular appearance, two of my vertebrae were crunched into wedge-shaped structures. Diagnosis: two vertebral compression fractures. Broken back.

Mental evaluation:

- oriented to person, place, and time
- dull, bland

The effects of the medication brought into sharp focus another fear: getting hooked on pain meds. I dreaded the pain ahead but couldn't bear the idea of not being fully aware and engaged with the decisions that were coming.

My less confident Linda persona knew that there wasn't much left of her body, and what was left had some pretty ugly scars. How could Dave find that attractive and sexy? My dreams of hiking the John Muir Trail, scuba diving, biking, swimming around the pier, and wearing my bikini to the beach were all gone. *Will I ever drive, make love, or work as a radiologist again?*

I was afraid of falling into a huge black hole and never crawling out again. Even worse, what would I do if Dave decided to walk out those double doors and never come back? I couldn't imagine life without him.

It was useless to open my eyes. When I did, white lights, white walls, and white bandages blurred into nothingness. Without anything to hang on to, my mind spun, jumped, and fell. I needed something to touch or hold, or at least something I could think about. From my hospital room in Austria, I escaped to Mexico.

~

It started as a relaxing beach camping trip in Punta Estrella, Baja, Mexico, and what should have been a short walk to meet friends for lunch in San Felipe. Skimpily clad in bathing suits, tennis shoes, and windbreakers, Dave and I strolled north up the hard-packed sand, holding hands. We were young, carefree, and in love. Crashing waves sparkled in the morning sun.

The atmosphere was intoxicating. I drew in a lungful of salty morning air as I shaded my eyes to see beyond the expanse of sand. "It's like the entire world is out in front of us—like I own the whole world," I said.

Dave took a deep breath, then let it out. His shoulders relaxed, and the corners of that sexy mustache slowly curved upward. With his thumb, he gently stroked the back of my hand and winked. *God, it's great to be alive!*

Lost in contemplation and conversation, we walked for miles. San Felipe, which we'd expected to simply run into, never came into sight.

Our pace slowed as the midday sun burned down, parching our lips and subduing our spirits. We had an ocean full of water but nothing to drink. Finally, a dune buggier came upon us. Before speeding off, he gave us one bottle of beer, which we nursed between us for the next hour. What was supposed to be a two-hour, five-mile stroll stretched into a ten-hour, twenty-mile death march through desert sands. Our fears escalated when we stumbled upon a set of human skeletal remains. A cold chill went up my spine, and the telltale tingling of a spike in adrenaline radiated through the tips of my fingers and toes. *We are lost.* I looked around and listened—sand and more sand. *Is this how they'll find us?*

After night fell, shivering in the dark, with no food or water, the heat of the day replaced by a cold wind, we knew we weren't going to make it to our friends. We had no choice but to turn around and face the long slog back to camp. The first tears fell silently; then I started shaking. I stopped walking and burst out crying.

Dave stopped and put his arms around me. "We can do this. I'll carry you if I need to."

With my head down, I concentrated on setting a steady pace as I struggled to see the ground through the darkness. One foot in front of the other while we talked about whatever came to mind. When we ran out of things to say, I started to sing and was surprised when Dave joined in. At first, we sang silly kid songs like "Old MacDonald Had a Farm," "Three Blind Mice," and "Row, Row, Row Your Boat." Then on to our national anthem and "America the Beautiful." Whatever we could remember the words to. We plodded on through the desert blackness and started to realize and appreciate each other's strengths: Dave the protector, Linda the entertainer.

It was the coldest, most miserable night of my life. As we trudged on, I relived each hour of the day and knew something had changed. The man I'd started walking with that morning had become someone I could trust with my life. We were strong. We were a team. He was my partner. I knew we could do anything if we did it together. I knew by the end of that weekend that we'd stay together.

I held on to that memory, mulling over it for hours—how Dave had put his arms around me in the darkness and said, "I'll take care of you. We're together." *Maybe he will stick around. Maybe this story is my beacon.* Rather than doubt him, I decided to be positive and try as hard as I could to make him happy.

What Kind of
Life Would That Be?

I am touched by her fear. She is mangled and crumpled and lies in an ICU bed with an amputation bridge over her from the waist down. But I know that she isn't really afraid of that. The pokes and prods and needle sticks by the nurses make her wince, but she really isn't afraid of those, either.

The future, which twenty-four hours ago was a happy family vacation in Bavaria, is now no vacation whatsoever. It looms large and will need to be dealt with. But she isn't afraid of that, either. Her mind will already have begun to figure out work-arounds for losing her right arm, as well as her legs, searching for a way that will allow her to practice radiology.

Death. She has no fear of that. And I know she has thought about death.

This is the first time we've seen each other. Alive. It is me. I am the source of the fear.

I am not angry. I am not menacing her. I am not remonstrating with her. I am just standing here, with the competing emotions of ecstasy over seeing her alive and anguish over why this happened to her causing tears to spill down my cheeks.

But I know that she isn't really afraid of me. The fear is that I might not have been able to stand there, and, more importantly, that tomorrow, next week, next month, or five years from now I will not be standing by her. The fear is that I will leave. She is not afraid of my presence. She is afraid of my absence.

But she is also afraid of constraining me, and that is what touches me so deeply. It is so thoroughly and genuinely Linda.

"I will understand if you don't stick around," she said as she squeezed my hand. Those were the first words I heard, not a wailing, tearful "Don't leave me!" Just a measured "I've been thinking about this, and I would understand."

A concern for my happiness, my future as a doctor, my desire to have a family, my love of an active, outdoor lifestyle resulted in her being able to glibly allow me to leave. No questions asked.

We are husband and wife; we are not new to each other. She has been making me a better person for more than six years. I stand touched to my core by that fear and by the way she has accommodated it.

Fuck this bullshit. I'm staying! my mind screams.

Will I miss her piano playing? Will I miss watching both hands fly across the keys while both feet race over the pedals of the pipe organ? Will I miss having her ride her Bianchi alongside me while I run? Will I miss the hikes in the mountains? Don't ask.

Will I miss having her climb, with bare feet, up onto my shoes so she can reach me with her lips and give me a kiss, a spontaneous gesture of love and caring that I have always savored? Will I miss having her right and her left arm looped around me for a hug? Will I miss gazing at her sexy, slim legs and the gentle caresses of her right hand? Don't let me think about those things. It hurts.

I am here, where I belong, and I am staying. Even if our lives are reduced to the simplest of activities, she can still be my sunset and I can still be her moonlight.

I have done a lot of thinking through the night as well, most of it recognizing the cruel reality that she might be dead by morning. I have dealt with her death and the prospect of life without her. To find her alive this morning is a gift beyond imagining, and I am ready to push on at her side.

"Olsie," I started, "let's think about it this way. None of my cancer patients, at the time of their diagnosis, know whether they will get better or get worse. Many do get worse, but they still fight hard. Your trauma was yesterday. You are not going to get worse. We are going to work and fight to make you get better little by little. My cancer patients do this. We can do this."

I know slow progress both from my practice and from my long-distance running. I have learned that even when you can't see the finish line, if you keep going, you will reach it. Concentrate on some small goal on the trail ahead of you, and then refocus on another small goal that allows you to go long and seemingly impossible distances without having to think about their magnitude. Running has taught me patience.

I am here. I am staying. I'm happy to be here, even though there is no finish line in sight.

Running to save her switched my soul into reverse. She had been making me a better person for six years. I knew I was a better doctor, a better man, and a better husband yesterday than I had been before we met. I hadn't done this to myself. Her soft and gentle influence had washed away and abraded some of my sharp edges, anger problems, and perfectionism. Her tolerance of me and my hard personality went beyond patience. It was her.

But she wasn't finished. There was still a lot of work to do. She owed me a lifetime of this. I wanted a lifetime of it. My soul was not ready for life without her. So I ran to her. My soul was ready to die beside her. So I leaped in front of the train to grab her and hold her. My soul wanted to be intertwined with hers from then on. Dead or alive.

This morning, my soul is not ready for life without her under any circumstances. Where would I go? And, most important, what kind of life would that be?

Fuck that bullshit! *my brain screamed again.*

So, here I am. I'm staying. There's work to be done, so let's get started.

CHAPTER 2:

The Pact

....

Post-op day two. Into the ICU swept a small, bony woman with chestnut hair gently sagging in a bun on the back of her head. Her thin lips were painted bright red, in contrast with her darkly penciled eyebrows. Her bronzed skin showed early signs of leathering, a trait we came to associate with Austrian and German sun worshippers.

"*Guten Tag*," she said curtly but with a smile. "I'm *Schwester*—Sister—Nora, and I will be your nurse. I am sorry my English is so poor. Do you speak any German?"

"No, I don't, but Dave speaks a little," I said, grateful to hear her heavily accented English words.

"The doctors say that you are stable. We will move you to another room."

Just two days after surgery, with IVs clanking and wheels squeaking, *Schwester* Nora and an orderly rolled my bed out the double doors of the ICU, down a hall, into an elevator, and out again, depositing me into a regular hospital room on the men's ward. Dave's room. The good news was that he was in the bed next to me. The bad news was that our beds were in a trauma hospital. It was time to start moving and learning to do things for myself.

~

After we were settled and the nurses left, I noticed a mirror lying facedown on the rolling bedside table. It was the kind my hairdresser might hand me. I stared at it, wondering what I'd see. There were already so many body parts lopped off, as if I'd been pruned. I desperately hoped my face would be normal: twinkly green eyes, dimples, impish nose, and even the freckles and moles I had previously tried to wish away. Now, feeling so small and egg shaped, I craved at least one recognizable aspect of my former visage. Screwing up my courage, I leaned over to reach for the mirror. Why didn't it move? And then I remembered. My right arm was gone. My favorite arm. The one that did everything automatically. The one that my brain was still sending messages to. I stared at the mirror for a while, acutely aware of the pain in the blunt ends of my amputated extremities. I felt as though I could reach out and pick it up with my right hand, but, of course, I couldn't. My right hand wasn't there.

I closed my eyes and felt tingling electrical sensations where my legs and arm used to be. I could sense my nonexistent legs bent at the absent knees, my missing lower legs and feet poking through the mattress toward the floor, just as if I were sitting in a chair. My departed right arm bent at the elbow, my hand slightly curved, resting relaxed in the neutral position. How interesting. It was as if these sensations were a safety mechanism, the products of a deceitful nervous system tricking my brain into thinking everything was as it should be, as though trying to forestall the inevitable distress resulting from so great a loss, delaying the dismal reality of being limbless. But if the limbs weren't there, how could this be me? How could I be alive? How could I be a person when the perpetual motion that had previously defined me no longer seemed possible?

I desperately wanted to look okay, for everybody to still see me as a person, a normal person. At this point, I'd settle for just looking normal from the shoulders up. I closed my eyes and wrapped the fingers of my left hand around the handle of the mirror, dragged it to the edge of the tray, and slowly raised it.

I cringed when I saw my reflection. My pale, haggard face, framed by medium-length, frizzy brown hair, still had scratches and scabs on it. But, worse than that, my right shoulder, freed from the weight of my arm, had floated up to take position next to my ear. With the mirror still in my left fist, I immediately pushed my wayward shoulder back down where it belonged. It stubbornly crept back up.

This was unacceptable. If I didn't fix this, I was certain that for the rest of my life people would see me as a lopsided egg. *I need them to see my face—a normal, happy face. I will make people respond to me by talking to them and smiling; my disposition, at least, is one thing I can control.* If my objective was composing a semblance of normality, step one would have to be taming the shoulder. *I can do this.*

Later that afternoon, Dave's family and his mom's best friend, Adrian, shuffled in, despondent and teary-eyed. They huddled at the foot of my bed, not sure where to look and struggling to meet my eyes. His mom, Donna, dabbed at her swollen, bloodshot eyes. His father who was usually talkative and demonstrative, fixed his gaze on the floor, face ashen, shoulders slumped in abject misery. Jack, who was driving at the time of the accident, already looked like he might never recover from this tragedy.

Anguish banished their usual sparkle. Their attempts to speak produced fragmented sentences so soft and tremulous the words were unintelligible. The fragility of my appearance—so divergent from that of the vibrant and intact young woman they used to joke about adopting should Dave ever end our relationship—left them faltering, unsure what to say or do. I suspected that in their minds' eyes, they were seeing me bikini-clad and pulling weeds in their backyard. Hugging or kissing this tiny remnant of me was, as yet, too much for them to attempt.

Adrian took charge of the emotional scene—a service she and her husband, Johnny, would perform countless times over the next year. Her sweet Southeastern drawl could go from comforting to commanding in a heartbeat, and it became part of the music accompanying my recovery. "Linda, how are you doing this afternoon? Have the doctors been in to see you? Are your bowels working yet?" Today I broke off the friendly interrogation, knowing it could go on interminably if I let it.

They stood with their arms wrapped around each other, unsure whether to accept my giggly, goofy smile, and joking banter as signs of good mental health or of denial and mild psychosis. Playing to the competitiveness I knew they all possessed, I challenged them to the first of many rounds of my newly devised distraction. "Hey, I've got a new game called whack-a-shoulder! First one to push my shoulder back down below my ear gets a kiss. Ready . . . go!"

That first night together since the accident, only three feet separated our beds, but Dave and I both felt the need to be closer to each other. He climbed slowly out of his bed, cautiously pulled down the sheet, and gently climbed into my bed. The warmth and strength of his body were simultaneously soothing and energizing. I didn't know what to do, so I cried. We were tired, but we wanted to hold each other and talk. Not about the bad stuff—there was plenty of that during daylight hours. I turned my head so I could see Dave's face: his lips and familiar mustache, his blond sideburns, and his green eyes.

I wanted to hug him, to feel his warmth and strength pressed into as much of me as possible, but I couldn't get my arm around him. Just changing position in bed was almost impossible. Without legs to extend, I couldn't roll over. Without both arms to push with, I couldn't sit up. I couldn't even wiggle. It appeared to me that my left arm would have to do the work of the three missing extremities. I grabbed the left bed rail with my hand and pulled. Nothing moved. Using my now precious left arm, I reached across my body to the right railing, grabbed it firmly, and attempted to haul myself up.

My shoulder lifted a couple of inches before a sharp jolt forced me to let go. Suddenly, my broken back demanded my attention. Since it was an invisible injury, it was easier to forget until I moved. Out of sight truly was out of mind. As the days went on, I would find that the agony of back pain overshadowed that of my amputation sites. Dilaudid was the only thing that subdued the torment for a few hours. And therein was another major mental battle for me.

I was petrified that I might become a narcotics addict. As I looked down the road into my future, I could see two outcomes. One was immediate relief of severe back and amputation-site pain. Something to make me feel good immediately and to push away all the issues that were facing us. Something that would let me smile and laugh and be worry free. The other was to figure out how to handle the pain mentally or physically to get through this immediate postoperative and hospitalization phase. To convince myself that even though it would be tough and hurt within the next few weeks, it would keep getting better and eventually go away. Going through this thought process, I was reminded that deep down I wanted to be in control of my life. I didn't want to take any chances that a drug could seize control.

And at that moment, we were in control of what happened next. With almost imperceptible motion, we leaned into each other, creating a cocoon between the railings of that hospital bed—a place where we learned to cuddle and love in a new way.

~

"*Guten Morgen,*" said Nora as she entered our room. One hand held a clipboard. The other rested on the pill arsenal she wore around her waist, a miniature pharmacy she was authorized to dispense based on her assessment of the situation—a system very different from the rigid doctor-prescribed, pharmacist-dispensed, nurse-delivered method in our hospitals at home.

I grimaced and broke into a sweat. *Oh God. I don't know if I can do this again.*

Mornings were filled with the customary doctoring and nursing activities of a hospital: eating small amounts of non-descript food; bathing and cleaning up; recording of vital signs and assessment of tubes, catheters, and medications. These mundane tasks led up to the barbaric, excruciating dressing changes that I constantly dreaded.

Dave hobbled, still in his cast, to the side of the bed opposite Nora and took my hand as she spoke in clipped English:

"How did you sleep?"

"What have you eaten?"

"When did you . . ." She searched for the word, then motioned toward the toilet.

"What of you hurts? How much?"

Between her English, Dave's German, and my emoting, all questions were asked and answered.

Satisfied that she had seen and heard enough, the fifty-year-old spinster decided on the painkiller or sedative of the day. Without ceremony, she unwrapped the foil pill package and gently but firmly shifted my body and shoved the medication up my butt!

"Dave," I whimpered.

He squeezed my hand and said, "It's quite efficient. Delivering medications rectally, rather than orally, is actually more successful, because many post-op patients are nauseated and throw up their pills, thereby making them useless for pain management. Administering it rectally is always going to be effective, unless you've got diarrhea."

"Well, I'm *not* nauseated, and it's as if she didn't know I have a mouth, which is fully capable of opening and swallowing pills of any size or shape," I said. "And it's so gross!" He patted the back of my hand.

It wasn't about efficiency or effectiveness. It was about the indignity of it all and the mounting fear of what was coming next.

Once the medication began to take effect, one of the surgeons and Dave would change the dressings. One or two nurses would assist them. Though they all worked quickly and expertly, I screamed as the dressing around each freshly cut and skin-wrapped bone was pulled away. My body reflexively recoiled from each touch, but with nothing to push against, I could only twist my spine and squeeze my shoulders, moves that brought fresh waves of pain and accomplished nothing but to tighten my hospital gown around my neck and expose my body. Each forty-five-minute session felt like a lifetime of agony. When they were finished, Nora would slip her hands under my armpits and situate me upright in my bed, my body swaddled in bandages, then slide her hand up my exquisitely tender right shoulder. Sometimes I screamed. Sometimes I was too exhausted to do even that.

Dave settled himself on the bed next to me as Nora herded the other staff members out the door. He was clean-shaven, and his scabs were healing, but the inner turmoil caused by the necessity of the dressing changes and the pain they caused me played out in his eyes. He looked at me for a long time before leaning in and gently kissing me on my sweaty forehead.

~

My family arrived on Thursday. There were no cell phones in 1979. They'd scrambled to gather passports and tickets and had gotten on planes, my parents on one and my siblings on another, knowing only what Dave had told them during the shattering call: I was on the critical list in the ICU. They arrived not knowing whether they would see me alive.

I knew how they would feel long before they arrived.

My dad, the textbook stoic pathologist, was devastated. I was his first child. The one who, as he did, played the piano and organ. The one who had followed him into medicine. He would be wondering how I could still be a doctor.

My mother, the talkative one, treasured and admired her oldest daughter with the bubbly personality and easy laugh, the one who craved constant activity and had a zest for adventure. She would be wondering if I could ever recover my joie de vivre.

My brother, Albert, and sister, Janice, who are one and a half and five years younger than I, respectively, were accustomed to my role as the bossy, strong-willed older sibling. Seeing me abjectly dependent was a striking change for them. They would be wondering how to reconcile this egg-shaped bundle of bandages with the vivacious, assertive sister they loved.

In my family's eyes, life as I knew it had come to an end, a very unfair end for someone who had so much going for her. I'd been a focused and happy child who studied and worked hard. While not touchy-feely, my parents had nurtured all three of us with their words: "You can be anything you want to be." They were strong people with a loving and supportive marriage, and they'd celebrated with me when I'd found a wonderful husband, someone they admired and respected. Even so, this was a huge blow. The kind that could tear apart even the strongest bonds. The kind that made you question God. Why would anyone want to believe in a God who would let *this* happen? This grief made it almost impossible to function—to lift your arms, to move your legs, to breathe, to speak.

Their grief might be something I could fix. In fact, I knew only I could do so. I had to greet them with a smile and show them immediately that even though I was still wrapped in bandages, recovery was underway. And Dave and I needed to prove unequivocally that we knew what we were facing and were already setting our plans in motion.

"Dad! Mom!" I yelled, as Jack and Donna led my parents into the room to see me for the first time. They hesitated near the door, trying to stand tall and strong for me. It didn't work. My mom sank into my dad's arms, tears streaming down her cheeks. They looked small and helpless. I needed to take control.

"Get your butts over here so I can give you a hug," I said.

They shuffled toward me, clinging to each other. Sitting up as straight as I could manage, I flung my left arm out toward them, a wide grin splitting my face in two. This would come to be my signature invitation for an embrace. "Come on, what's taking you so long?" We leaned into each other as they reached the side of my bed. I didn't let go for quite a while.

In my peripheral vision, I could see Jack standing in the corner, almost as if he were trying to shrink out of sight. Dave and I were worried about this first encounter between our parents. I hadn't seen Jack smile since we'd been in the hospital. Knowing we'd need their love and support for the rest of our lives, we realized we had to set the stage right now for our families to stay strong and united. They would need to see us succeed in order for that to happen. If I could start the minute they saw us, we'd set the tone for all our future interactions. *I can do this.*

"Hey, how do my shoulders look?" They looked at each other, then back at me.

"What? What are you talking about, Linda?" my mother said.

I flashed her a smile. "Well, I'm lopsided now, 'cause my arm's gone, so I need everyone to remind me to keep my shoulders even."

My dad stood tall and mute at the foot of the bed, taking it all in. When Dave and I burst out laughing, they looked totally confused. From tears to the loony bin. What a roller coaster we put them on. But we had caught them off guard. Momentarily distracted from tragedy, they had to smile at our goofiness.

"Mable and Albert," Dave said, "the military has a room for all of you at the BOQ in Garmisch-Partenkirchen. It's where my parents and Adrian and Johnny are staying."

"When word got out that two active-duty military members and their spouses were in a train accident, food and support started pouring in from every direction. Everything's covered for you while you're here," I said. "I'm so glad you're with us."

Having crept despairingly into our hospital room, my parents had a glimmer of hope in their eyes when they left us late that afternoon. *We can do this.*

⌒

By now, there was a full-blown battle going on in my head, one of David-and-Goliath proportions. One side was manned by troops saying, *Don't open your eyes . . . don't move . . . cry a lot . . . moan and groan . . . be a pain in the butt . . . make everyone miserable and feel sorry for you . . . why me . . .* The other side was peopled by forces cheering me on:

Open your eyes . . . look around . . . smile . . . talk to people . . . laugh . . . pretend everything will be fine . . . make everyone around you feel good . . . you can do this. The fighting was fast and furious.

Just when I'd convince myself to be positive and open my eyes, I'd see the gaping space on the bed where my legs should have stretched out in front of me, with ten toes that could wiggle on command. That would make me slam my eyes shut in avoidance.

I'd always been an upbeat person, and I wanted to stay that way, no matter what it took. Attitude was the only thing I had control of, so my mind went into overdrive trying to be optimistic and cheerful. I pretended my brain was a muscle, which, if squeezed tightly enough, would power my way through all the challenges ahead of us. I wanted the open-your-eyes team to win in the warfare going on in my head. *I can do this.*

An unwilling captive in a hospital bed, I had plenty of time to start working this through. I found myself looking for things to surmount. It was like an addiction: give me something to work on, something to think about, ways to start replacing what I'd lost. This helped me, but I also wanted everyone around me to take heart and see things working out for us.

Later that day, a nurse walked in holding her fist next to her ear, a pretty good international signal that there was a phone call for us. Dave got out of bed more quickly than usual and followed her to the nursing station.

A phone call. Just the distraction I need!

He returned quickly and, with help from the nurse, put me in a wheelchair. The phone was on a long cord, but it reached only as far as the door to our room.

"Hello?" I greeted my mystery caller eagerly. When I heard my best friend, Juli, on the other end of the line, I automatically continued, "What are *you* doing?" This was, and still is, my signature start of a phone conversation. Knowing that it was an expensive international call, we kept it short. As we came to the end, she said, "It's so good to hear your voice. You sound just the same."

"Of course I do. I *am* the same—just a lot smaller." I was grinning from ear to ear as Dave pushed me back to my bed. Hearing a friend's voice gave me a new infusion of hope and confidence. I knew we needed a whole team of people to help get us through this. I knew we would have help as we returned home. *We can do this.*

"We are going to learn how to do things with your left hand," Nora said as she walked into my room a few minutes later. She placed a small, unopened milk carton on the tray in front of me.

"Open it!"

After turning it over several times, I gripped it with my teeth so I could rip it open.

"*Nein, nein!*" Nora admonished. "You must not use your teeth. Never, never!"

Despite her abrupt bedside manner, Nora was far from a cold practitioner; she was a do-what-needs-to-be-done-to-get-better kind of medical professional. Dave called her our angel. I had to agree. Her personality and style suited us perfectly.

Winning the imaginary good-patient award became my goal, so I busied myself by turning the carton every which way, hoping it would just open itself. No such luck. Spreading apart the triangular top wasn't too hard. I laid the carton on its back and used the tray table's counterpressure. But if I opened it like that, the milk would spill. When I set it upright and tried to open the seal, the carton slid away from me. I pulled it closer, ignoring the throbbing pain in my back and trying to keep the ends of my legs from banging the bed's side rails. As I hunched over the carton, my shoulders tensed up, inching closer and closer to my ears.

No matter what I did, the glued surfaces would not part.

My tiny body shrank into the bed, knowing I was a failure. An endless black tunnel stretched into eternity. *How will I live if someone has to do everything for me?*

David, zero; Goliath, one.

"Dave," I blurted out that night, "I need to have a hysterectomy when we get home."

"What?" was his incredulous response.

"Well, it would eliminate having periods, so one less thing to learn: how to use a tampon with one hand. Plus, I'm not sure having kids is a good idea."

He jumped up. "Hold on. Don't make rash decisions."

"Why? I've been thinking about it, and I don't think it's fair for kids to grow up with a disabled mom like me."

I'd already decided it would be a crime to give birth to children who would hate us for making them part of a family with a mom who was in a wheelchair, who couldn't do things with them, and who looked funny.

"You've gotta be kidding. Don't I have any say in the kid decision?"

To be honest, I hadn't considered Dave's feelings on this matter, so I wasn't prepared for his answer.

"I want to have kids. And I want them to be your kids," he said.

"But—"

"When they get to be teenagers, they won't like us anyway, no matter who we are. They'll think we're dinosaurs. And there's no difference between being disabled and being a dinosaur."

Immobilized by my healing amputations and compression fractures of the spine, I spent most of my waking hours focused on learning to use my left hand: tearing toilet paper off a roll, cutting food, turning the pages of a book, holding the book open, taking the cap off a pen. Nothing in my life could I take for granted.

One afternoon after lunch, a nurse brought in a toothbrush and tube of toothpaste and left it on the hospital tray in front of me. Hunching over to hide what I was doing, I glanced around furtively, then bit the top before anyone could reprimand me, "Don't use your teeth, ever." The teeth marks left in the screw cap would give me away. *Well, they are absolutely stupid to think that I can do everything with just one hand!*

With shaky fingers, I squeezed the toothpaste tube and watched with dismay as the toothbrush wobbled over onto its side, smearing the tray with a white, gooey mess. Every inanimate object seemed to have a life of its own. Things that used to sit still now teeter-tottered, swayed, or rocked and rolled in front of me.

I couldn't open a milk carton or squeeze my own toothpaste, much less take care of my bodily functions. The pain pills constipated me, but my bladder still worked. After my catheter had been removed, I had to be lifted up and put onto a bedpan. When the nurses insisted that I try to move my bowels, they would put my arm around their shoulders and lift me, positioning me on the commode. Moving my back and the accidental jarring of the ends of my legs, or even touching them, made me want to scream.

Pain is one thing, but the worst thing in the world for me was needing help with these bodily functions. The stink from constipation. The poop, the pee, and, most awful of all, my period. It was humiliating.

"Dave . . ."

I don't like this. I don't like this. I don't want anyone . . .
"I'm staying," he insisted.

Did I want him to do it? No. But did I need him to do it? Yes. I knew that it was better for him to do it than to have anybody else do it. He protected me from other people having to be there and forced me to suck it up and get used to it.

Being physically stable was one thing. It was time now to turn our attention to our mental health, first to figure out what the big issues were going to be and then how we would solve them. That is not a very long sentence, only thirty-one words. But it signifies a huge project that would consume us for a long time. In fact, it would be years before we would know whether it had worked. It wasn't always a pretty project. In some ways, it helped that we were Dr. Linda and Dr. Dave, Patient Linda and Patient Dave, Wife Linda and Husband Dave. It allowed us to assess and respond to our situation in ways no one else could. We needed to identify problems as *we* saw them, not as others perceived them. In doing so, we unintentionally alienated people along the way.

One afternoon, after I'd been bathed and my hair washed, Adrian—who'd come immediately from Stuttgart, organized everyone's lodging, and acted as a liaison between our families and the military—stepped in once again to help. Everyone knew how much I hated my curly, frizzy hair, so she started blow-drying it to straighten it. "*I'll* do it!" Dave told her abruptly. The subtext was *We don't need your help.* She handed him the hair dryer without saying a word. Her cold expression said it all.

And when my aunt and uncle, who were traveling in Europe at the time, called to say they were dropping everything and flying to Salzburg to be with us, Dave told them he didn't want them to come, that we had plenty of people, and that he and I wanted to start taking care of things on our own. Looking back, I think we could have been more gentle or politic in our reactions. We were flailing to right a ship that had capsized and that would sink fast if we didn't take hold of it to keep it afloat. More people would only add weight.

~

"I feel like an egg. I'm a mess. How can you still like me?" I asked Dave as he carefully wrapped his arm around me one night.

In my brain, I was young, attractive, and sexy. There, I had an unending number of ways to entice Dave, but this tiny, legless, one-armed body in a hospital bed couldn't possibly seduce a young, hot-blooded male—especially a handsome doctor with a limitless future ahead of him. There'd be no more playing kneesies, no more standing on his feet to dance or reach up to kiss him, no more bear hugs. How would I keep his feet warm at night? There wasn't even enough of me left to cuddle with. How in the world could we ever make love again? Why would anyone want a sexless marriage? What would a virile, healthy young male see in my egg-shaped body?

"Olsie, you're more precious to me today than you were yesterday," he said. He stroked the curve of my body and buried his face in my hair. "I'm right here. I'm not going anywhere."

~

The hospital room was quiet and peaceful. Late-afternoon summer sun dappled the walls, and soft air came through the balcony door. All our family members and friends were gone, the surgeons had made their rounds, all the medical procedures and dressing changes were done, and we were alone together.

It was a time of day we had come to savor, a time when we could talk, hold each other, and then talk some more. And we needed to do a lot of talking and holding.

But at the moment, I was propped against the headboard, supported by two big white eiderdown pillows. My right shoulder was swathed in white Kerlix gauze. A white amputation bridge protected my lower torso.

"Can we talk about the afternoon of the accident?" I asked. Tiny beads of sweat formed on my forehead. I was dressed in only a hospital gown, but I was always hot.

Dave hobbled over and sat on the edge of the bed. He took my hand and replied, "Yes, what about it?"

I started slowly. "Dave, I know exactly what happened on the train tracks. I never lost consciousness."

"I know," he said. He dropped his head slightly, and his hand tightened around mine.

I chose my words carefully and continued. "I can't help but think about it all the time. I'm not sure how to feel about it. . . . And I'm not sure what we should do about it."

"You have every reason in the world to be angry. I'm willing to do whatever is best for *you*." I could see his anger and confusion.

"I know it wasn't intentional," I murmured, "but I'm not sure whether I can disguise my resentment."

"I understand," he responded. The weight of what I said seemed to rest on him.

I'd thought about it for days, but saying it out loud was somehow more difficult than I'd expected. *What if I change my mind? What if it comes out anyway? . . . Just say it!*

"What has happened has happened—nothing can change it. I want to do what's best for the future of our families. Who knows? You want to have kids. . . . We'll need everybody in both our families to help. We can't waste our energy on blame and anger."

Dave looked up and met my eyes. We both swallowed hard. This was our crossing of the Rubicon.

"It's your call," he said, stroking my fingers. We wiped our tears, and then, for the sake of our friends and families, present and future, with a kiss on my forehead, he sealed our pact: "We were in Berchtesgaden, Germany, when the van *stalled* on a railroad track."

CHAPTER 3:

A Room with a View

....

In August 1979, the Salzburg Festival was in full swing. Herbert von Karajan was directing a new version of Giuseppe Verdi's *Aida*, and the famous opera and symphony director Karl Böhm was directing his last opera at age eighty-five. A quarter of a million people filled the concert halls and outdoor stages for more than two hundred performances of symphonies, plays, and operas. Every hotel was sold out. There was no room at the inn, except at the Unfallkrankenhaus, the trauma hospital where Dave and I found ourselves in a second-floor, two-bed room.

The view of the beautiful, romantic old city contrasted with that of our sterile, austere room. From our balcony, the timeless charm of the Old Town stretched out before us as Dave and I straddled two worlds. Inside the sparse, utilitarian hospital, we were starting over, with grueling work ahead of us. Outside, picturesque Salzburg beckoned us to dream of the beauty that still surrounded us if we were just willing to reach for it.

"Hey, Linda, your shoulders are even. Good job," Adrian said as she approached.

Yes! Progress.

"We brought you some dinner," she said.

"A very special dinner, a dinner for two," Johnny said. He held aloft a covered dish, as if presenting a sacrifice to the gods.

"But before you eat these little guys, you've gotta know the story." He paused, as if for permission to proceed. "Now, the best way to find *Schnecken* is to set out on a forest path early on a Sunday morning with sturdy shoes, a walking stick, and a plastic bag. Keep your eyes peeled for these critters slithering along the path. Make sure you carry a *Schneckenring* so you know whether they're big enough to take and keep. The last thing you want is *Der Waldmeister* to arrest you for poaching." He had a twinkle in his eye.

"On a Sunday, huh? Not Saturday morning or Thursday afternoon? Sunday. Sunday morning?" Dave teased.

Johnny laughed and didn't skip a beat. "I take them home and dump them into a large, heavy-lidded crock, where they stay for a week or ten days, feasting on cornmeal, sweet white German wine, and herbs. What a life! When the purification is complete, we boil them in a large pot with more wine, herbs, and water. After they cool, I pull them out of the shell and rinse them. Meanwhile, we boil the shells, saving them for presentation when we eat them. To serve, you warm the stuffed shells, place them on little escargot trays, and serve them with melted butter, fresh bread, fruit, and cheese."

"Which we have right here," Adrian said as she pulled a loaf of bread from a local *Bäckerei* and several Tupperware containers out of her shoulder bag.

I squealed and without thinking tried to clap my hands

together. The sudden movement and momentum sent me listing starboard.

"All right, help me up, someone. I can't eat like this. I'm just grateful you took them out of the shells already. Nora would insist that I find a way to hold the tong in my left hand while using the fork with something else—something, *anything*, other than my teeth!"

We all laughed. Johnny set the dish down on the bedside table and pulled my high, cane-backed wheelchair over toward the bed while Dave gently scooped me up and set me in it. "My lady, may I escort you to your table?" he said.

"Yes. Please do. I'd like a view, please, something with a breeze, if you can," I said, using my most aristocratic voice and better-than-thou face.

"We have just the place," Dave said. He wheeled me through the sliding glass door, which opened onto a tiny balcony just big enough for a small table and two chairs.

The magic of the evening overpowered us. Below was a grassy area with large shade trees, walking paths, and a small gazebo. Beyond, the stunning view of the Hohensalzburg Fortress captivated us. Its massive whitish walls fade into a tan patina. Crenelated towers flank the corners, and small rectangular windows march along the tops of the walls, breaking the sameness. It consumes all the space on the largest hill overlooking the Old City. Adding to the charm are nearly a dozen delicate spires of old churches that rise to the base of the fortress. We felt like a king and queen that evening, looking over the city while the centuries-old fortress compassionately held vigil over us.

We gazed at this mesmerizing fairyland every day, letting it transport us to a place where everything was serene and happy. The undefeated citadel on the hill gave us strength.

Evenings became our special time together. We had no energy to waste on pity, regret, or anger. Exhausted but anxious to create our new normal, we primped, smoothed the bedsheets, and settled in with each other by nine o'clock. Someone had brought us a copy of *The Winds of War* by Herman Wouk, and its recently published sequel, *War and Remembrance*. Each had more than a thousand pages of war, romance, and intrigue, with enough historical accuracy to bring it to life for us. The sex scenes made me blush and cast furtive glances at Dave. I wondered if we would ever feel those things again.

One afternoon, Donna and Adrian sashayed into our room, giggling like schoolgirls. Adrian dangled a pretty wrapped box over my bed.

"Looky here," she teased, holding it just barely out of my reach. "Come get it."

I scooted toward her an inch at a time, reached out without tipping over, and snatched it away from her. "Ha haaa," I said. "Guess I showed you!"

Feeling a little smug, I dropped it on my lap, then realized I'd have to untie the bow, remove the string, undo the tape, and get the lid off. I snuck a look around the room, making sure a commando nurse wasn't watching, grabbed the ribbon with my teeth, and pulled. Voilà—out spilled a dainty set of white eyelet-lace baby-doll pajamas—the kind that shows lots of bare skin and cleavage.

I didn't know whether to laugh or cry. I held the skimpy top at arm's length and waved it back and forth. *Oh, heck— why not!* I jiggled my boobs free of my hospital gown and tried pulling the top over my head. The little straps hung on my ears. I wobbled precariously, trying to jab my left hand into the armhole. Dave was at my side almost instantaneously, gently tugging it down over my shoulders. Before I could stop him, he fondled my boobs and planted a loud smooch on my cheek.

The elephant in the room couldn't be avoided. Someone cackled; others averted their eyes. I had no idea how or if that was going to work in the long run, but at least, for the time being, he was acting interested.

The sexy pj's became my signature look.

By the end of the first week, everyone in the hospital knew who we were. The most glaring reason was that we were always speaking English and they were always speaking German. Our families had relatively free rein to come and go as they pleased. Nurses would linger longer than necessary in our room, and I'm quite sure we had more than the usual number of doctor visits during the day. Maybe the "free rein" was because of our language differences and we just didn't know any better. But maybe it was because our independent, adventurous American spirit made us somewhat of a delightful distraction.

At the end of every day, our families found their way back to their quarters at military housing in Berchtesgaden, emotionally exhausted. There were usually ten or eleven people: Dave's family, my family, and Adrian and Johnny. They were the grateful recipients of a steady supply of homemade food that arrived frequently from the military base in Stuttgart. Johnny's commanding figure opened the bar early every evening, and in his infinite wisdom he titrated the evening's gin and tonics as he felt necessary.

I'm told it was my dad who first suggested that they dance. He and my mom had been taking ballroom dancing lessons for the past few years and enjoyed practicing to big-band music on the tile entryway of their home in the evenings before dinner. We had grown up as strict Seventh-day Adventists, a religion that disapproves of dancing. This departure from our upbringing had been rather momentous a few years earlier. I can imagine my father standing up and stepping into the middle of the room, beckoning my mother, who of course would demur at first but finally hold her arms out to him as they came together for a romantic waltz or a fox-trot or maybe even a little cha-cha. I'm sure Dave's parents and Adrian and Johnny were quick to follow. Anxious faces tentatively smiled, then laughed, and then maybe there was even a chorus or two of Frank Sinatra or Peggy Lee.

One night, after a few of Johnny's "stiff ones," they got down to business and created a society to record and track the progress of my recovery. I'm still amazed at the name they came up with. They must have gone around the circle and asked everyone for a word to incorporate into the title.

From:
The Society for the Serendipitous Restoration of Social, Scientific, and Sexual Scintillation Among the Amorous, Erotic, and Occasionally Erratic Emmigrants [sic] to the Bavarian Barracks in Berchtesgaden

To:
The Famously Fantastic, Fabulously Realistically, and Resolutely Responsive Regenerates Confined in a Cozy Corner of the Krankenhaus

Greetings:
Having duly considered cautiously the characters of the confinees in question with the definite difficulties that developed, undoing (temporarily) the doings of the most durable doers in the domain of diabolical diagnostic designers, the Society awards the meticulous marks in management measures initiated by the ingenious ingenue and her consort in commodiously comfortable Krankenhaus cohabitation.

Bertchesgaden University for Mature Students
"BUMS"

Every afternoon, our families and friends straggled in with time weighing heavily on them. This seemed harder in some ways on them than it was on me. Their helplessness and my need for fresh air gave me a mission.

"I can't stand it in here anymore," I blurted out one afternoon. "I've got to get out of here! Let's find a way to get outdoors before I go stir-crazy."

"Great idea, Olsie!" Dave said.

The next time Nora stepped into the room, we pleaded with her to help us make a plan. "Do you think you could find a wheelchair for Linda so I can take her outside for some fresh air?" Dave asked.

She swung around and said, "*Nein*, you can't push her out there. You need to be in a wheelchair, too!" And with that, she swept out of the room. Five minutes later, she returned with another nurse and two cane-backed wheelchairs.

"Okay," she said to the other nurse. "On the count of three, let's lift Linda and put her in this wheelchair. *Eins, zwei, drei.*"

I clenched my fist and squeezed my eyes shut, hoping I wouldn't scream. They put me down gently and wrapped me in a snowstorm of white sheets and blankets. Dave settled himself into the other chair, a brown hospital robe over his hospital gown. Off we went on our first wheelchair adventure. Hospital fashionistas, we made our way down to the ground-floor lobby.

"Do you see what I see?" I asked as we neared the lobby gift shop.

"Uh, yes. Flowers, cards . . ." And then he did a double take. "Beer? Are they selling beer in a hospital lobby?"

Suddenly, we had a plan.

When everyone arrived that afternoon, we loaded up books and blankets. Adrian and Dave's brother and fellow accident survivor, Mark, rolled our wheelchairs down to the lobby where we bought a few bottles of beer and then paraded out to the garden. From then on, we held court outdoors every afternoon in the warm September air smelling of cut grass and happiness. Some days there were up to seven people, all of us taking turns at playing the role of jester. We tried to outdo each other with jokes and funny stories, becoming more ribald as the afternoon shadows grew longer. My goal was to make everyone laugh and see the future as full of possibilities.

My surgeons, having seen Dave show that he'd had plenty of surgical experience, happily allowed him to be doctor to me when they weren't around.

"My, you're healing up nicely, ma'am. No more catheter, no more IV," he said with an impish smile one morning after my doctors had made their rounds.

He went about his work. After a few minutes, he said what had obviously been on his mind the entire time. "And your boobs are perfect. Your bottom's perfect, too. You're still a turn-on."

"Doctor, I don't believe your behavior is appropriate. What *would* the hospital administrator say?" I responded coyly as the back of his arm "accidentally" slid over the thin fabric separating my boobs from his body.

"I'm just being friendly," he said with an unapologetic grin.

It sounded good. It felt good. But it was still hard to see myself as sexy Linda. Playing doctor was one thing. But Dave played nurse, too. He attended to my basic bodily needs and administered medication, for the most part, by suppository, the Austrian-German way. Those images were hard to shake and replace with the way things had been.

But that night, after everyone had gone and all was quiet on the hospital floor, he became husband again.

I watched from my bed as Dave, still in his cast, hobbled around the room, doing some tidying. He caught my eye and stopped at my bedside, leaned over, and kissed me softly on the lips. It felt good. Really good.

"Mmm, let me touch you," he whispered.

"Are you sure?" I asked. "Are you sure you want to? How can I possibly turn you on?"

"I've been dying to for days," he responded.

I smiled and let out a giggle before the reality set in. "Well, okay, but I don't know what will happen," I said.

"You're neurologically intact. Let's see what's going on with the supratentorial part, shall we?" he whispered.

He kissed me gently on the lips, carefully reached his hand under the sheet covering my lower torso, and found the sensitive area. He was soft and gentle and slow and patient and found that the sensitive area was just as sensitive as it had always been. After a few minutes, I moaned softly, and all the tension of the past ten days left my body in one exhale. We were lovers again.

"Mmm, that felt so good," I murmured after a few minutes. "But what about you? I can't do anything."

"Don't worry about me. I'm fine," he said. It was clear to see that that was a lie! I smiled and winked at him—a small consolation prize, but all I had to offer.

"And we just proved that you are, too, so I can wait. But I will make you pay me back when you can. You're going to have a pretty large accounts payable by then!"

"Ooh, okay," I said, giggling. "I'll look forward to that! You better be ready."

A little friendliness had crept into the Salzburg trauma hospital. That night in bed, wrapped around each other as much as two people with three good arms and one good leg between them can, we sighed the collective sigh of partners climbing back up the steep cliff from which we'd been so unceremoniously thrown.

In the second week of our recovery, a petite, young, blond occupational therapist walked in one morning and introduced herself.

"*Ich heisse Sonja. Wie heissen Sie?*"

By that time, I had an automatic response to anyone who came into our room speaking German. I'd flash my big smile and say either "*Guten Morgen*" or "Hi, how are you?" It didn't matter which, because as soon as I said it, indecipherable German words flew out of their mouths, and all I could do was up my smile a notch and shrug my shoulders.

Responding to my *Help me!* look, Dave jumped in. "*Guten Morgen*, Sonja. *Wie geht es Ihnen?*"

Then he turned to me. "Say, '*Ich heisse* Linda.'"

She smiled expectantly at me as she placed a pencil and piece of paper on the bedside table. She took out another piece of paper and showed me a list of words. With gestures and pointing, she indicated that she was going to dictate them to me so I could write them down.

"*Der Hase*" (the rabbit), she said in a slow, deliberate voice.

I gave her a confused look.

We laughed as I tried to pronounce each word on her spelling list. I failed the German vocab test, but I assiduously practiced writing them every day.

As had become our routine, when the hospital quieted down in the evening, we shifted into work mode to grapple with how to re-create our lives. Dave took charge and made things black and white. We shared our fears and frustration, but he went a step further and made me put pen to paper and write a list of the issues we were facing.

"Hon," he said one night, "yesterday I asked Adrian and my mom if they'd bring us a notebook and something to write with." Reaching into his nightstand, he pulled out a tablet and notebook and limped over to my bed. "Which would be easier for you, a pen or a pencil?"

Pen or pencil . . . I don't even know how to hold a stick in my left hand. How can I even make this minor decision? I opted for the pen. *Maybe the words I write will be stronger and come to life.*

Where do you start when you have to start all over at age twenty-nine? Can you categorize your life in a list on one page? How many words does it take?

Looking back at the pages we saved from those nights, I see the answer. The first page has ten categories: Personal, Rehabilitation, Professional, Social, Marital, Family, Psychological Adjustment, Sports Activities, Occupational Adjustments, Desirable Goals. The words tilt up and down on the page in my second grade–looking print. Four more pages provide ideas and details about how we might proceed in moving on with our lives. They are poignant in retrospect, the result of much soul searching at the time.

"I'd like to send a postcard to the White," I told Dave one morning.

The White Memorial Medical Center in Los Angeles was where I was doing my radiology residency. This was my first attempt to reconnect with my career.

Like magic, a pen and postcard of the Mozartplatz appeared on my hospital bed stand. Even though I'd been practicing for a couple of days, my left hand fumbled with the pen. *Should I hold it with three fingers or four? Where should my thumb be?* The edge of my hand covered most of the postcard as I tried touching the pen to it. *How am I supposed to write and keep this stupid little card from moving around?*

"Can you bring over that coffee mug and set it on the corner of this card?" *This is downright hard, if not impossible, but I can't imagine someone holding things for me the rest of my life. So come on, Linda—just get over it and figure it out.*

09-02-1979

Dear Rad Gang,

I couldnt [*sic*] have found a prettier town to have been incarcerated in. They have let me look at my X-rays before and after. They'll make an excellent teaching file. This is one of 6 hospitals in Austria for trauma only. We've had exellent [*sic*] care. You can all do us a big favor by finding the best rehab cent and prosthesis [*sic*]. Love, Linda

The first three words run up- and then downhill: "Dear Rad Gang, I couldnt [*sic*] have found a prettier town to have been incarcerated in." I choke up a little as I start. I try to make it sound positive ("prettier town") and make fun of it ("being incarcerated").

My childlike handwriting continues: "They have let me look at my X-rays before and after. They'll make an excellent teaching file." Every radiologist in the country knows what a teaching file case, or TF, is: radiographic images that show something unique, or classic, or difficult to diagnose. Teaching file cases are fascinating to look at but are almost always bad news for the patient. My X-rays were certainly worth the proverbial thousand words. Then again, you don't need to see my films. The diagnosis is visible to the naked eye.

"This is one of 6 hospitals in Austria for trauma only. We've had exellent [*sic*] care." *This is really weird—I can't spell.* It is shocking to write a sentence and discover that several words have letters or whole syllables missing. I forced myself to spell the words out loud and then squeeze in the missing ones haphazardly. I hadn't given a thought about how to spell these simple words since I was in second grade.

It'd been many years since I'd given a thought to many things. Suddenly, I was forced to rethink everything.

"Be careful. Don't let them psychoanalyze you."

Mal Braverman, MD, was a psychiatrist from Beverly Hills who had been doing research on burn victims in the Unfallkrankenhaus. A tall, husky man, he'd introduced himself by saying he'd heard a lot about us. Dave and I liked him immediately. A warm, friendly person, he spoke with us for about an hour. I described the accident, telling him I'd been conscious the whole time. Together, Dave and I told him our deepest feelings and worries, and shared the plan we'd put together for the future. He questioned both of us. Psychiatrist questions. He watched and observed us.

"I'd say both of you are handling this problem just fine. No doubt it will be tough. I'm pleased to see how well grounded you are and what you're doing. When you get back to the States, they will want both of you to undergo counseling and analysis. Don't let them dig into you, because I know they'll want to go into deep, Freudian-type psychoanalysis, and neither of you needs that."

We were stunned but pleased and promised to take his advice. It had been only two weeks since the accident, and I'd had no nightmares or panic attacks and was not reliving the accident. But, having no experience with the mental consequences of trauma, we were unaware of the potential for long-term sequelae. Unbeknownst to us, the *Diagnostic and Statistical Manual of Mental Disorders (DSM III)* was being revised to include the change from "gross stress reaction" to "post-traumatic stress disorder" and was evoking a lot of attention. Dave and I were strong individuals, and deep down we felt that if we combined our strengths, we could work through this as a team.

"Ahem," Johnny said. He held himself up straight like the commanding Navy officer he was, demanding the attention of the court.

The breeze blew through the trees, and had it not been for my disfigurement and bawdy attire, it would have been easy to mistake our party as a group of tourists enjoying a secret garden tucked in a fold of the ancient city. In many ways, we wanted to stay, but it was almost time to go.

"May I have your attention, please?" Johnny continued, theatrically snapping a sheet of paper in front of him. "The Society of Sexual Serendipity presents to you, Dave and Linda, your Report of Progress!"

Our families and friends guffawed as they took turns reading aloud their assessment of our recovery.

0 = Outstanding; **E** = Excellent; **S** = Satisfactory; **F** = Failing

Achiever	0	Knowledgeable	0
Borborygmic	E	Odiferous	F
Cursive Writing	S+	Passionate	**Oh, Oh**
Defecation	S-	Quiet	F
Exhibitionist	E	Resourceful	0
Flatulating	S	Sudoriferously Sexual	0
"Gutsy"	0	Temptress	**0++++**
Horny	**Oh!**	Urination	**S (F- as of 9/2/79, 12:45—you fail!)**
Irrepressible	0	Virtuous	**F+**
Juvenile	S	Warm (Ich bin)	0
Kissable	0	X-rated	**0, often**
Lovable	0	Terrific	**!**
Manner (Bedside)	**NA**	Ze END	**?**

Our last night in the Salzburg hospital came in late September. Five doctors filed in and stood at the foot of our beds to bid us an emotional farewell. Three and a half weeks earlier, these vastly experienced, gray-haired, stern trauma surgeons had saved my life. The one who was fluent in English spoke for them.

"We have something we'd like to say. We've been watching you for the past three weeks. If you were Austrian, you might not have opened your eyes yet. You have shown us what we believe is the American spirit."

Dave and I were silent, not wanting to break the spell. We knew it was time to leave the Unfallkrankenhaus and our castle on the hill, which had brought us deep fear and magical hope. By then, I knew that Dave's love would give me the power to prove these men right.

Six weeks short of my thirtieth birthday, I found myself strapped to a gurney in a back room of the Salzburg airport. Dave stood next to me, holding my hand, the only one I have now. We felt naked. We were leaving the trauma hospital where we'd been for three and a half weeks. Our hands were free of luggage, but our minds were full of baggage. We were going home, back to what we knew, but everything was unknown. Breathing was the only thing left that was automatic.

I was a baby, tiny, no clothes, beginning a journey on which I must start over, learn a new way to do everything, from sleeping on my side to dressing to sitting in a wheelchair, and to getting people to see me, notice me, know me.

We were silent. There were no words for where we were. Even though our minds overflowed with questions and fears, we knew it would do no good to verbalize them. *It is time for me to grab hold of myself and take charge*, I thought. At the same time, I knew that I must let Dave hold me and take care of me until I could do things by myself again—*if* I could ever do anything by myself again.

Through the large plate-glass windows, I saw the tarmac stretching away from me, vanishing. At intervals, planes roared in and throttled off. Nothing stays still. Everything is coming or going, and while the passengers inside them think they know their destination, I wondered how many of them, like us, would not end up where they thought they were heading.

CHAPTER 4:

(In)dependent Wife

A hot, dry Santa Ana wind greeted us when the door of our Navy medical transport plane opened at Naval Air Station Miramar late on the afternoon of September 20. Waves of heat rippled across the tarmac as four muscular Navy corpsmen hoisted my litter and carried me down the stairs into the blinding sun. Dave and I were silent as the military ambulance drove us to the Naval Regional Medical Center San Diego emergency department, where a young, blond female intern assigned to do my admitting history and physical met us.

She was so beautiful that I couldn't stop staring at her. I shrank into the gurney. *I am a doctor, just like her, but no one is ever going to think of me like that again.* I closed my eyes and hoped she couldn't see me crying. My side of our conversation was a series of mumbles.

She pulled her stethoscope out of her white coat pocket and asked, "Can you sit up so I can listen to your heart and lungs?"

I fumbled with the sheet, trying to pull myself up. Nothing moved. Likewise, my attempt to roll over failed. I gasped when she lifted my gown and placed her cold stethoscope on my bare chest. She winced and averted her eyes when she saw my mangled body. I imagined myself soaring out the window, fluttering away with normal arms and legs.

As we rolled toward the admitting area, I held Dave's hand. This was his hospital. Mark had been born there twenty-five years before, and we'd been married in the naval chapel less than two years before. There were already emotions tied to this place.

Out of nowhere, Dave asked, "Did you know that this was the largest military hospital in the world during the Vietnam War?"

"Really?" I said, more than anything just to keep the conversation going.

"Yeah, it had over twenty-five hundred beds at that time. Now we have twelve hundred."

That's huge by any standard. *There must have been miles of hallways. I bet people got lost all the time. How would you keep track of everything in a behemoth like that? How many X-ray machines would have been there?* Dave has always been a master at knowing when and how to distract me.

The next morning, bodies in neat white uniforms crowded into my room. Having been a medical student and resident, I recognized the ritual of daily morning rounds and understood the pecking order. The chief resident stood at the head of my bed and shuffled a handful of three-by-five-inch notecards. The scribbles on each were there to remind him of the pertinent facts for the patients in his care. The other residents, medical students, and nurses whispered while checking their notes for the relevant lab and X-ray reports.

Voices floated back and forth above me. "This is a twenty-nine-year-old dependent wife who was admitted last night by medevac from Salzburg, Austria." Dependent wife. *Dependent wife—that's what I'm called in this hospital. Just someone married to an active-duty military member, not a person. In my hospital, I'd be called Doctor.*

"She and her husband were in a train-versus-car accident in Berchtesgaden, Germany, with traumatic amputation of both legs above the knee, a right-arm amputation, and L3, 4 vertebral fractures. Surgical sites are well healed. Her husband, Dave Hodgens, is an active-duty physician, third-year resident here in Radiation Oncology." I recognized and appreciated the detached-sounding clinical description summarizing my condition as something I'd done many times over the past several years. But now that I was the "she," the description didn't compute. I thought they must be talking about a different "she" until I looked at the empty space in the bed where my legs should have been.

The intern pulled back the sheet and touched the large red, puckered scars that extended over the ends of my residual legs, what they called *stumps*. He tugged on the shoulder of my hospital gown to display the wrinkled, flabby remainder of my right arm, which ended at my shoulder.

I saw them looking over and around me. *I'm a nobody, a crip, a patient who appears to have nothing ahead of her but life in a wheelchair.* I stared up at the orthopedic team. *They don't know that I'm one of them, that I'm in the third year of a diagnostic radiology residency in Los Angeles, that I passed part one of my radiology boards just before leaving for Germany. They don't know me as a person yet. I'm just an interesting case. After all, what are the chances they'll ever get to work with a triple amputee again?*

It was difficult to smile when my broken back hurt like hell, and I had sporadic spasms of pain in my nonexistent feet or hand. Pain that I eventually learned is called *phantom pain*. Pain that jabbed and stabbed me unexpectedly and for no good reason. Pain that hurt so badly that sometimes my entire body would jerk violently. I felt it most often at the outer aspect of my left foot—or where my left foot should have been.

I was always in pain, always hot and sweaty. My face was pale and gaunt, my hair frizzy and unruly. *What do they see? Certainly not the attractive used-to-be me. Not the five-foot-five-and-one-half-inches-tall, well-proportioned, 103-pound me.* They were looking at a three-foot-tall, egg-shaped thing that weighed seventy-five pounds. I closed my eyes. *I'll ask Dave to bring in a picture of us together so people can see the real me. Maybe one with me wearing a bikini or my tight jeans and halter top. Maybe a picture of Dave hugging and kissing me, so they'll know that I was attractive and sexy.* I had wished for such pictures when we were in Salzburg.

I wanted—needed—to show them that on the inside, I was still a normal person.

Determined to sit up and be part of the conversation, with a little butt jump, I reached with my left hand for the trapeze bar that hung from a large orthopedic frame over my bed. Grabbing the bar lifted me slightly off the bed. But without the aid of legs or another arm with which to push and pull, I couldn't brace myself. My body swiveled, and, embarrassed, I let go of the suspended bar and fell back onto the pillow.

"Is she ready to be fitted with prosthetic legs? What are our options here?" the attending orthopedist asked.

Dr. Webster was in charge. I liked him. Dave liked him. But most important, he was hell-bent on rehabilitating me.

Dressed in their crisp white summer uniforms, the interns and residents glanced at each other. "Some studies show that stubbies are psychologically beneficial because the patients are upright immediately," one resident said.

"What are stubbies?" I asked.

Finally, someone acknowledged me.

"Stubbies are short prostheses without a knee. They attach to the stump and have a rocker-bottom platform in lieu of a foot. They're useful in the post-op period to get people upright quickly, help strengthen them, and keep them from developing hip contractures."

Stump. Why would anyone say that? It sounds like something you'd hear discussed at a lumberjack symposium. Why can't they just call them my residual legs?

"Why can't I just have regular-size legs?"

"This is quick. It's easier and takes much less energy to walk. And you're probably not strong enough yet to use long legs."

None of these orthopedists had ever seen a triple amputee. It was September 1979, only six years since the end of the Vietnam War. The wave of six thousand amputees from that war were treated in one of six military hospitals when they returned stateside, but San Diego was not one of them. So, in a way, we were all on the same learning curve.

As the doctors moved on to the next room, I tried to imagine myself with fake legs. *Will I ever really walk again?* I've since learned, from various doctors and medical journals, that it takes 280 percent more energy for a bilateral above-knee amputee to walk with prosthetics than a person with normal legs. According to a 2007 article in *inMotion* called "Stepping Up to Health, Using a pedometer for amputee fitness," if you were to follow the recommendation to walk 10,000 steps per day, I would expend the same energy after only 2,500 steps. Only 20 percent of bilateral above-knee amputees become successful prosthetic users. I can't even find any numbers for the success rate of triple amputees.

The magic of Salzburg was gone. No longer could Dave and I gaze out our window and see the Hohensalzburg castle floating above us. No longer were we the darlings of the Unfallkrankenhaus, the brave young American couple whom our Austrian doctors and nurses admired.

An inaccessible bathroom beckoned from across the room, its doorway too narrow for a wheelchair to enter. Oh, to be able to stretch, sit up, and leisurely swing my legs over the side of the bed, then stroll into the bathroom and sit on the toilet in privacy. Instead, I jabbed the buzzer and commenced the long wait for an overworked orderly. When he arrived, he leaned over my bed, put his arms under my tiny torso, and pulled me up against his chest while I hung on like a monkey. He walked the ten feet into the bathroom and lowered me onto the toilet.

"Let me know when you're done," he said. Then he walked out, leaving the door wide open.

Eventually I learned to transfer myself onto a bedside commode, an alternative that was only a little more acceptable than calling the orderly. It's like having an open-air toilet in the middle of your living room. Over the next two months of hospitalization, I would spend hours agonizing over whether I really needed to have a bowel movement.

When I finished, I pushed the call button and sat helplessly until he came back to reverse the process. *Reasons number one through ten for me to learn to walk are so I can go to the bathroom by myself.*

In the dark hours of that evening, I tried to be positive about my goals. I forced a smile, but my wet cheeks and quivering voice betrayed me. Reality eclipsed my shining positivity. Anger consumed me.

"Why did this happen to me . . . to us?"

Dave cuddled up to me as I sat on the hospital bed, one of only three places I could be: in a hospital bed, on a toilet, or in a wheelchair.

"If I could have just run faster, I'd have gotten you before the train hit."

As our tears flowed, he whispered, "Remember our pact." Putting his arms around me, Dave assumed the role of cheerleader. "Olsie, our lives aren't over, you know . . . we can still go out to eat, go to movies, work . . ." He hugged me tightly.

"And we *can* have a family. Even if you don't have legs. Even if you can't walk."

By the time Dave left each night, I was exhausted.

Falling asleep was easy. What I couldn't do was *stay* asleep. Most nights, I found myself in a twilight zone of dreams, reality, and memories. I fought to find stories of fun times, anything to get through the dark, lonely nights. Incarcerated in my hospital cage, I would drift into fun-filled, physically active outdoor sequences. I'd ride my mint-green Bianchi racing bike twenty miles, with a gain of 3,300 feet, into the San Bernardino Mountains. Lured by the apple orchards and cinnamon–apple pie fragrance in the bakeries of Oak Glen, I'd ferociously pump up steep, windy roads with hairpin turns, then speed back down to Redlands, tucked compactly over my racing handlebars. Or I'd cruise leisurely along the long, empty two-lane stretches of San Timoteo Canyon Road, deeply inhaling the sage and dirt aromas of the chaparral hills and rocky canyons.

I'd jerk back to no-leg reality when I woke and lie there confused by the dreams that always seemed more real than what I saw when my eyes were open. I began to understand schizophrenia, delusions, and hallucinations, the inability to know which scenes are real.

During our stay in Salzburg, I kept telling myself that I was a doctor. When we got to San Diego, I started reminding myself that I was a radiology resident and that I needed to get back to my residency. But even after Dave brought my books and stacked them within reach of my bed, I'd open one and flip through a page or two before putting it back down. Telling myself I was a doctor was one thing; actually being one was another.

Dave marched into my room one morning while I was picking at my breakfast.

"You ready, Freddy?" he said.

"For what?" I mumbled, my mouth full of cold, rubbery scrambled eggs.

"Today's the day for your cute little ass to get to work down in PT."

My cute little ass had no desire to be rolled anywhere, let alone to what was probably a stinky hellhole in a Navy hospital basement.

Five minutes later, we stopped outside a room labeled PHYSICAL THERAPY. The door opened into a large square space filled with exercise tables, free weights, chin-up bars, and floor mats. It could have been any gym in America. Except for its clientele.

Light streamed through windows that stretched all the way around the room near the tops of the walls but didn't reach into the souls of many of its inhabitants. Near the door was a beaten-up institutional-gray metal desk strewn with loose papers and patient charts, around which lounged three or four burly Navy techs. Three women in white uniforms chatted over coffee. One looked to be several years older than me. Two appeared to be my age. Insignia on the black shoulder boards of their uniforms indicated they were officers, but as a civilian I was clueless about their ranks. The warm, muggy air smelled sweaty and mixed with the odor of alcohol and antiseptic.

I took a deep breath. *No use pussyfooting around.*

All seventy-five pounds of me sat up straight and gripped the armrest of the extra-wide wheelchair that Dave had pushed me in from my hospital room down to Physical Therapy. My nondescript white T-shirt and gym shorts made me fit right in with the other patients in the room, except they were all guys who were much younger and much bigger than I was.

"Pardon me," Dave said firmly to a woman wearing what were, unbeknownst to me at the time, commander shoulder boards. "This is my wife, Linda Olson. She is here for a physical therapy evaluation." He was also dressed in Navy whites, his shoulder boards informing them that he was a doctor and a lieutenant commander.

All three women turned toward him and then, in unison, looked down at me. While one shoved papers around on the desk, looking for my orders, I swiveled sideways in my wheelchair and put my hand out toward the woman standing closest to me. After a noticeable pause, she reached out with her right hand. In a split second, using a maneuver I'd already mastered, I rotated my left hand 180 degrees to meet her outstretched palm so she wouldn't be embarrassed by awkwardly connecting with my left hand.

"I'm ready. What shall we do?" I asked, with a big grin on my face. "Or maybe I should say, what do you think I can do with only one arm?"

They just stood there. *Okay*, I thought, *let's do something*.

Commander White sighed and cleared her throat. "Your orders came down yesterday."

The other two women fidgeted, gazing down at the floor, or their shoes, or whatever else they could find to look at. Anything but the thing sitting before them. Silence. I'm not sure who was more uncomfortable.

"You've been assigned to Lieutenant Donna Pavlick, whom I believe you met the other day," she said as she handed the chart to one of the women. My eyes followed the chart to the hands of the young woman I'd spoken to briefly in my room. She was about my age, with medium-length blond hair. About the size I used to be. And a no-nonsense look. I was the first to throw down the gauntlet.

"I'm ready. Let's see what we can do."

Now it was her job to help make me strong enough to walk with prostheses. She, like everyone else there, had never seen a triple amputee, but I was soon to find out that she had a will equal or superior to mine.

Dave and I followed her to a corner of the room, where he leaned over, put his arms around me, and set me up on an exercise table.

"The accident was four weeks ago, in Germany. We just got back here a few days ago," he said.

"I'm tired of lying in bed. I need to get started on doing something," I said, feigning enthusiasm and butting into Dave's conversation.

"Are there any open wounds?" Donna asked as she took off my JOBST stockings and felt the ends of my legs to assess how much muscle the surgeons had been able to wrap around the ends of the bones after they'd been cut away.

"Did they skin-graft anything?" she asked. She was all business.

"No," I said, before Dave corrected me by saying, "She has a split-thickness skin graft on her left medial thigh."

"They were meticulous surgeons," I continued, grabbing center stage again. "All my wounds were totally healed by the time we left Austria. We had incredibly good medical care there, probably better than we'd have gotten many places here in the States."

Satisfied with my level of healing, my new therapist looked away from my legs and motioned toward my torso.

"Okay. The most important thing for you will be core strength, so can you lie down and do some sit-ups?"

"Sure." I lay down on my back with my hand behind my head and crunched up, or, shall I say, tried to crunch up. Nothing happened. I tried again, with the same result. My short legs flew upward, but that was it.

"Here, let me hold your legs down, and you try again," Donna said. Not much better.

The three of us sat side by side on the table, letting the

gravity of the situation settle in. *I have to make this work so I can walk again.* I looked at Dave. *I have to do this so he can stop feeling guilty.*

Donna stood up. "I've never seen, let alone worked with, a triple amputee. And I'm pretty sure there's no book to follow. I guess we're on our own."

So, three twentysomethings set out to create a plan, work their butts off, and hope for success.

My goal was to get Donna to laugh; hers was to get me to concentrate.

It was game-face time whenever my wheelchair rolled into the big PT room. With a loud "ta-da" and a boob jiggle, I'd make my grand entrance every morning and every afternoon. After all, a gal's gotta do what she's gotta do when she enters a room full of young sailors. The room was full of train wrecks like me, so I figured anything went to get people to look up and laugh. "Laughter is the best medicine" was my motto from day one, an approach that works wonders when people are allowed to make fun of the shitty things that have happened. Without legs, I couldn't sashay in or wiggle my butt, so I perfected the boob jiggle. Before long, everyone developed their own risqué greetings. But for all the innuendo, I was one of the guys.

"Hey, Linda," shouted a young guy in a wheelchair one afternoon. "How many pull-ups are you going to do today? Bet I can do more than you."

"Yeah, right. . . . I have to do only half of what you do, 'cause I have only half as many arms as you."

"She got you, bud," came a response from another corner of the room.

I butt-walked onto the large exercise table and rolled onto my stomach. I was intent upon mastering one-armed push-ups. It was hard. Really hard. In fact, I wasn't sure I could do it.

I looked around the room. My eyes lit on a skinny kid who couldn't have been more than eighteen years old.

"Hey," I said, looking straight at him. "What's your name?" He looked away, ignoring me. But I was relentless. "Why don't you come over here? I need some help figuring out how to do these stupid push-ups." Before I could count to ten, I was surrounded by guys stretching out on the table, one arm behind their backs, showing me their own versions. The physical therapists and techs sauntered over to goad us on for a bit before breaking up our lovefest.

~

It took a few weeks for me to hear the story of how Donna and I got paired.

The Monday after my admission, my request for an evaluation had arrived in Physical Therapy.

As usual, Donna read through the orders and stacked them for assignment. She admitted later that, knowing how much work my rehab would be, and deep down questioning her abilities, she'd stacked this pile so that Mel, another therapist, would draw me.

Before Mel finished reading it, she started crying. "I can't do this one."

"Why not?" a tech asked.

"No way. It's a doctor's wife. Plus, she's a new amputee," she sniffled.

"She's probably fat and whiny. I don't want to get near her. I bet she'll make us all miserable."

At that point, Commander Weber walked in, took a look at the papers, and turned toward Donna.

"Miss Pavlick, you'll take the amputee case. You're the most experienced."

Pairing me with Donna turned out to be one of the most

important elements of my rehab and long-term success as a functional, walking amputee. Her younger brother had been injured as a preteen, with resultant brain damage and severe physical impairment requiring long-term care, which she and her family had provided at home. Teaming up with me seemed therapeutic for her in ways that I couldn't understand for a while.

Stuck in my bed, I'd pretend that the hospital's green walls were at the White Memorial Medical Center in Los Angeles. *That's where I should be. My legs at their walk-run pace, rushing from room to room, doing upper- and lower-GI barium studies under fluoroscopy, dictating chest X-ray results, calling referring docs with exam findings, being grilled at conference by my radiology faculty.* I'd completed the written portion of the American Board of Radiology exam just before the accident. I should have been studying for the oral examination that all radiology residents take at the end of their residencies. *Only nine more months, and I should be certified by the American Board of Radiology as a diagnostic radiologist. And then, finally, after twenty-three years of school and training, I should be getting a great job somewhere, and Dave and I should be able to think about settling down, having a family, and eventually growing old together.*

I looked at the thick radiology textbooks stacked on my nightstand, books Dave had placed there, hoping I'd start looking at them. I didn't have the energy to pick them up, let alone study them. On the other nightstand sat a fourteen-by-seventeen-inch radiology view box, the hallmark of a radiologist at that time. It had been placed there at the request of Dr. Webster.

As the weeks wore on, Dave started pushing me downstairs to the radiology residents' noon conference—an important educational part of every residency program. I fought him at first because I didn't want the guys I knew to see me—guys I'd studied and attended conferences with. Dave eventually won that fight, and, by extension, I won, too.

As I sat between a bunch of Navy men in white uniforms, my cotton T-shirt and shorts made it look as if I'd just popped in from the beach. Sometimes the on-call radiology resident would come up to my room to look at interesting X-ray cases on my view box with me or take me down to the department to read films in the evening for a while. Because I was in my last year of residency training, I had more experience than many of them, and they liked having a more experienced set of eyes look at the cases with them.

I guess Dave thought that if I looked as though I'd just come in from the beach, I might as well actually go.

"Hey, Olsie," he said one evening, "I'm trying to get a weekend pass to take you home Saturday after PT and bring you back Sunday night. Let's go to the beach this weekend."

"Wow," I said with a big smile. "That would be very cool."

Saturday arrived, and Dave pulled out my bikini and put it on the bed. I looked at it and said, "I am *not* going to sit on the beach in a skimpy bikini and let people see me looking like a freak."

"Oh yes you are," Dave said. "I'm going to parade down the hill to the sand with you in my arms. I'm going to show everyone how beautiful and sexy my wife is! And I don't *ever* want to hear you say again that you look like a freak."

Squirming and grumping, I did my best version of a poor, ugly, wimpy wife refusing to cooperate. I was getting stronger, but I lost what had been a full-on battle.

After pulling into the parking lot, Dave said, "Hang tight. I'm going to take our stuff down and will be right back up to get you."

"It's not like I'm going anywhere," I mumbled.

I watched as Dave sauntered down to the beach with two folding chairs under one arm and towels and a beach bag in the other. People glanced at him as he passed, just another good-looking California dude out for a day at the beach. Nothing anyone hadn't seen before. *That's about to change.*

When he lifted me from the car, I hid my face in his shoulder and squeezed my eyes shut. I felt the ground beneath us change from pavement to soft, deep sand. I didn't open them until he finally leaned over and plopped me into my low-lying beach chair. He smiled and took off my long-sleeved shirt and shorts, leaving me in my bikini. I just watched as if I weren't in my body. *I have a book to read. I can look at the Scripps Pier and the waves. I can turn and face Dave and pretend I'm having a good time for his sake.* Over the next few minutes, I did all three and finally gave him a weak smile that said I was actually glad to be there and grateful to him for making me do this. As I did, I pulled his face down to mine and gave him a big kiss.

When I let him come up for air, Dave reached into the bag and said, "Come on—want to play a little Frisbee?" Clearly, he'd planned this whole thing to get me back doing some of the things we used to do, to prove to me that we could still do them, just a little differently.

In the hospital, nothing changed. Every time I woke up, I still looked like an egg. Less than ten inches of my upper legs remained, and there was nothing where my right arm should be. What was left was so little that I looked tiny balancing in a wheelchair. Day after day, it was the same oppressive horror.

It wasn't the train hitting the van.

It wasn't seeing my foot and my leg and my arm.

It wasn't anything I'd seen in the past. It was about what I could see in the future.

Losing life as I knew it.

Losing my husband.

Losing my looks, my career, my identity.

At least going home with Dave on weekends gave me some sense of normalcy, some sense of security.

~

"All right, Dave. Let's see how these things work," I said one Saturday afternoon after strapping on the stubbies I'd been prescribed. "Lift me out of this chair, will you?"

Dave lifted me out of the chair and placed me down on the floor. And I mean way down. Fully upright, I was only forty-eight inches tall. The distance from my crotch to the floor was probably about eighteen inches. To walk, I had to hike my hip up a little, move my "stump" ahead two or three inches, come down on the rocker-bottom platform, and then repeat it on the other side.

My hand nearly dragged on the floor.

"I look like an ape!" I looked up at Dave and thought, *When in a wheelchair, I view the world from belt level. Now, with stubbies, I'm at crotch level! Strapped in, trapped in. What a choice this is, looking like an egg or tottering around on mini stilts.*

A flood of tears followed.

"Olsie, listen," Dave said as he bent down to look me in the eyes. "Just try a few more times. It's better than being in a wheelchair, isn't it?"

Not by much.

Shuffling was all the stubbies were good for. Because I had only one arm, I couldn't pull myself up into or safely lower myself out of a chair. I couldn't climb up onto the toilet. Nothing in the kitchen was reachable. Sweeping the floor and a little gardening were possible. But I would clearly never make a living wage.

"I can't do this, Dave. Other people might like them, but I *hate* these things! It's humiliating."

While I recognize the advantages of putting bilateral above-knee amputees into stubbies as early as possible to prevent contractures, build strength, do basic activities around their homes, and get exercise, it didn't take long for me to push what I thought were useless objects into the back corner of a dark closet.

Butt-walking was my only other option. It's still often the best one. I do this by getting down on the floor without my prostheses, putting my residual legs straight out in front of me, and moving forward one butt cheek at a time. At my size, I advance 4.4 inches with each butt step. Sometimes I put my hand down on the floor and push myself a little with each step. This increases my stride to nine inches.

While this is a good way to get exercise, it pretty much makes me the human equivalent of a snail. It makes Los Angeles traffic look like a race. On the upside, it's a good way to clean the floor.

"This is a waste of time," I told my doctors the following Monday. "I'll do whatever it takes to be fitted with full-length legs. Let's get on with it."

The ortho-rehab team gave in and wrote a prescription for my first full-length pair of legs.

My prosthetist, Randy Strong, explained in mechanical jargon what needed to be done to create my first set of long legs. I paid little attention to the details but did hear him say we needed to supply him with a pair of shoes. Finally, a girlie thing we could do!

Sensible, sturdy shoes with leather soles and flat or small heels, he'd instructed. So, off went Dave and his good friend Lee Parmley, yukking it up as if they were still college boys and out to conquer the world.

"We looked at every pair in the store," Dave said expectantly when he returned. I lifted the lid of the shoebox. Inside were two utterly atrocious brown pilgrim shoes with big, flat square buckles on the toes.

"Uh, are these for me?" I asked, trying to keep a straight face. "They're old-lady shoes. I can't wear these things!"

"But they look like they'll be stable. We don't want you falling," Dave and Lee said, almost in unison.

Stable shoes. My new reality. What happened to cute shoes or sexy shoes?

"Never send a man—or, worse, two men—to do a woman's job. We're taking these nasty things back. *You're* taking *me* to take these things back and find some that I can be seen in."

We giggled our way into the shop and returned the pilgrim shoes. I sat up straight as they pushed my wheelchair up and down the aisles, peering intently at dozens of shoes before settling on a pair of leather slip-ons.

"Why don't you try these on?" the salesman said as he handed me a size 8. We all burst out laughing as I dangled it with my one hand, hovering over the nothingness at the end of my foreshortened lap.

I loved getting everyone to laugh at my disability. This was something I wanted more of.

~

On October 16, nearly seven weeks after the accident, Dave and I were in my warm, stuffy hospital room, watching the 1979 World Series on our new nine-inch TV. The Pittsburgh Pirates had evened up the series by winning game six against the Baltimore Orioles when Randy walked in carrying *the legs*. Like some medical pied piper, he was followed by nurses, therapists, and doctors, who jostled for space in my room.

These medical professionals were truly invested in my

rehabilitation. I think they realized that trauma is no respecter of persons, that they could have been in my place. They seemed amazed by Dave's absolute commitment to me and our marriage. I think they wondered whether they would stick around if they were saddled with a loved one's unexpected lifelong disability. After all, we live in a disposable society. We throw out the Bic pen when it runs out of ink. We buy new shoes rather than resole our worn ones. We leave when things don't go our way.

Randy placed the legs straight out on the bed, the open ends of the sockets up against my residual legs.

I reached down and ran my hand along one's rigid socket and over the thick felt strap screwed into its top. The sockets were glued to a boxy knee contraption that bolted into naked, hollow metal pipes, all of which ended in the brown slip-on shoes I'd chosen for myself.

As everyone watched, Randy said, "Okay, Linda. Here's how these work." He pulled from his lab coat a pair of long cotton stockings and showed me how to pull them all the way up each of my legs and then push up the rigid sockets so the rims reached my pubic bones. He crisscrossed the thick felt straps tightly over my pelvis and fastened them around my waist.

"Well, this is the least sexy garter belt I've ever seen . . . but I *love* it," I said with a giggle. There were a few muted chuckles, but everyone seemed anxious to see how they'd work.

Dave turned me gently so the legs dangled over the edge of the bed. I put my arm around his neck.

"Dave," I whispered, "can I really do this?"

In a voice so low no one else could hear, he said firmly, "You can do it. I'll help you."

"Are you ready?" Randy asked as he and Dave slipped their hands under my armpits.

I nodded.

"Okay, Dave . . . one, two, three." I heard sniffles as Dave and Randy hauled me up onto the stilts.

The first thing I saw were Dave's green eyes. Something was wrong. I was looking straight into them instead of up into them. *They've made me too tall!* Then I glanced down to see if maybe the legs were tan. *How cool would that be? Tall and tan, like the girl from Ipanema.* They weren't, but ahhh, what a relief.

Ahhh turned to *ugh* and then *ouch.* The bony ends of my legs hit the bottoms of the sockets. The inner, upper socket ledges cut into my tender skin and pushed against my pelvic bones. Randy and Dave helped propel me three or four steps. The clumsy experiment lasted less than two minutes before I crumpled in a sweaty heap on the bed.

The staff were all pleased with themselves as they strolled effortlessly out of the room. They'd made a Linda stand-up doll, which meant they'd done their job. I watched them walk away, leaving to go home, where they could run, skip, jump, wear cute clothes, walk on the beach, and live carefree lives.

The truth was that I was exhausted. My legs hurt. The positive was that I now knew I could look normal because I'd have legs. But they hurt so much that I didn't know if I'd ever be able to walk. Dave and Donna were more positive than I was.

I waited until Dave was gone, then burrowed my head under the pillows and cried myself to sleep and to dream. Vivid Technicolor dreams. Dreams with real legs and two arms.

Dave's day consisted of running in the dark early morning hours, then driving to the hospital, coming upstairs to see me, and then going back down to work in the Radiation Oncology department in the third basement of NRMC. When finished, he drove home to do household chores and then drove the eleven miles back to the hospital so he could spend an hour or two with me, watching baseball or football, before I fell asleep.

I, too, had a rigid routine:

Get up.

Eat breakfast.

Go to PT.

Back to room for lunch, collapse, and nap.

Return to PT.

Return to room.

Eat supper.

Visit with Dave.

Turn off light, go to sleep, and dream.

Dream every night that tomorrow morning my legs and arm would be where they belonged and I'd go back to finish my radiology residency, go on vacation, get a job, have a family, love Dave forever. Be normal.

Every morning, I considered whether I wanted to get up or bury myself under the pillows and cry. My stomach churned; my eyes squeezed shut; my breathing was shallow and rapid. But I did not bury my head. I did not cry. Every morning, I turned on my iron face.

Dave and our kids still recognize it: the face that says, *Leave me alone; I will do this.*

I continued the interminable PT that consumed my life. Two or three times a day, I was pulled into the leg sockets and strapped onto the stilts. My white gym shorts offered some level of modesty, hiding my underwear and everything else from the general public when I moved. In my opinion, what they saw was much more grotesque than anything that was hidden: fat, lumpy-looking, hard, skin-colored sockets that encased my "stumps;" a metal knee joint plugged into the bottom of the socket; a shiny, hollow aluminum pipe that extended from the knee into a rubber foot cut flat through the ankle. My shoes looked truly out of place on the contraptions.

At least my core and supporting muscles were getting stronger, thanks to Donna's creative, if brutal, therapy regimen.

"Linda, it's time to start walking, really learning to walk, with your new legs," she said one morning.

Sweat rolled down my face and my curly hair frizzed as I stood for two minutes, then three, then four. Clutching the parallel bar with my left hand, I tried to lift one leg and put it back down. Donna stood behind me, holding on to a wide leather belt she'd strapped around my waist. If I fell, I wouldn't fall far.

Dave was there every day, sweating with me.

"Remember, it takes a baby a year to walk. Give it time!" he'd say.

When frustrated, fearful tears would start to flow, he'd repeat his mantra: "I didn't marry your arms and your legs. If you can do it, I can do it."

He asked a million questions, wanting to understand everything Donna and I were doing so he could do it for me if he needed to. I started moving. Not sure if you'd call it walking, but it was movement.

Meanwhile, we did our due diligence and obtained second opinions from other rehabilitation centers. "You will not be able to walk from the parking lot into a grocery store, because it will take too much energy," said one well-known rehab doctor. "It will be nice to have legs for looks, but you will need to use a wheelchair to go anywhere."

Another said, "Triple amputees can't ambulate successfully. It takes too much energy, and they all give up."

The third looked at us and said, "I don't know, but you're young enough, and you may be motivated enough, to make it work." Amid enthusiasm like that, we thought it no wonder there were not very many successful walkers out there.

"Okay, Linda. We'll show them. You *are* going to walk a mile." With that challenge, Donna mapped out a walking course for us, one with benches or chairs at close enough intervals that we could rest frequently. I went out onto the hospital grounds, tethered to my physical therapist by a rope and belt around my waist. People saw me. I kept walking. Some said hi. Most looked away. In my mind, I said, *Hey! I'm just like you. In fact, this could be you!*

Every day we made progress. Every day we walked farther than the day before. Step by step by step.

Soon, the toy-soldier *thump, thud, thump, thud* became my trademark sound. *Thump* when the knees locked and *thud* when the heel struck. The belt came off. A quad cane provided enough support that I could walk on my own. I was free!

As I walked on my own, I looked people in the eye, smiled, and said, "Hi, how are you?" I forced them to look at me and respond. No more talking to belly buttons and crotches from a wheelchair for me, and no more letting people act as if I wasn't really there.

Four months after the accident, I walked a mile in my new legs.

Life as I knew it had seemed to be over. But was it? Are we defined by our legs? What do we do when we get new legs? Are we the same person? A new person?

I wondered, if I gave it my all, where it would take us.

Cry My Eyes Out

I'm in Rose Canyon in San Diego, crying my eyes out. I do this every day. It's a cool October morning. Dawn is about an hour away, but I know this place so well that moonlight and the company of stars are all I need. I'm running on dirt roads where nothing but tall weeds and bunny rabbits exist.

This is my safe place. I'm alone and free to let all the emotions work themselves out without shame. No holding back. Why her? My thoughts turn from sorrow and anguish to anger and become absolutely homicidal. I let the anger run full force through me. It drives my legs faster. I know I will forever have the energy of this anger to push me.

By the time I head back to the house, the eastern sky has started to gray. The tears have dried. I know that my legs and lungs have done their work and that my tensions are calmed. I can now think better and plan. I will now be able to focus my concentration and direct my energy toward her problems and toward those of my courageous cancer patients—problems that, in the grand scheme, are far more important than mine. As I cool down, take a shower, and put on my uniform, I reach a peaceful equilibrium that will last until tomorrow morning.

CHAPTER 5:

Climb Every Mountain

....

I squeezed Dave's hand and nuzzled his neck as I whispered in his ear, "I can't wait! Can you believe we're doing this?"

I kept looking up at the arrivals-and-departures board to make sure our flight from JFK to Frankfurt, Germany, was still on time.

It had been only nine months since our last trip to Germany. Just nine months since the accident. Nine months learning how to walk on my clunky fake legs. Nine months through a yearlong medical leave of absence from my radiology residency at White Memorial Medical Center in Los Angeles.

Thankfully, the radiology department at UCSD had welcomed me with open arms, allowing me to observe as a nonpaid resident so I could get back into the learning process. While I'd gotten strong enough to walk a mile in my strap-on legs, Dave's legs had become even stronger. Carrying me up and down the stairs several times a day was part of his daily routine. His legs did double duty. It was a good thing he was young and I was lightweight.

"Dave, did you hear that?" I asked, poking him in the ribs. Our flight was announced in English and then German. Hearing the guttural words made me tingle with excitement. I was a giddy passenger. I've always loved people-watching in airport terminals, parading down long jetways, climbing the stairs, and walking sideways down the skinny airplane aisles, looking for my seat number.

But mixed with my excitement was nervous energy that made my body shiver.

We would be spending a couple of days with Dave's parents, who were still stationed at Patch Barracks in Stuttgart, then would travel by train on to Salzburg and Venice. We'd brought my one-arm-drive wheelchair but had optimistically decided we'd leave it in my in-laws' Stuttgart apartment and do the trip to Salzburg and Venice without it, hoofing it like any other young couple in love. We intended to prove that even though we might look funny, our lives were nearly normal and we could still have a good time.

The nine-hour Lufthansa flight was exciting at first. I giggled and snuggled up to Dave after we buckled our seat belts. Following dinner and a glass of wine, we settled in for the long haul over black nothingness thirty-five thousand feet above the Atlantic Ocean. But as the hours dragged on, I started squirming. My residual legs were swelling inside the tight sockets of my prostheses, and I felt welts starting to form along their tops. I reached down into my jeans and tried to wiggle the skin around to relieve the pressure. My skin would blister and break down if I didn't get my artificial legs off soon. If that happened, our full-week trip would be ruined.

Dave's slow, rhythmic breathing told me he was already asleep. Not wanting to wake him, I sat thinking. And then I became aware of the pressure building in my bladder. I sat motionless, trying to ignore it. *Nope. That's not gonna work. Need a distraction.*

I reached into the gap between my body and our shared armrest, pulled out my book, and skimmed a few pages. *If I could just take off my legs and if the flight attendant could just hand me a catheter . . .*

When Dave finally squirmed a tiny bit, I poked him. "Please," I whispered. "I need to go to the bathroom—really badly."

"Why didn't you say something sooner, hon? Of course," he said.

Dave unbuckled his seat belt and stood up. Positioned awkwardly in the narrow aisle, he leaned over and, as if I were a limp doll, pulled me into a standing position. As the plane lurched, he used his body to brace me. I wriggled sideways down the narrow aisle, holding Dave's belt as he walked in front of me.

We'd both flown many times, so we knew that airplane bathrooms are tiny, but as he opened what looked like a trap door into the mouse house–size lavatory, it was clear right away that my peculiar method of sitting down wasn't going to work in this teensy space. To sit on a toilet, I had to find something stable behind me that I could put my left hand on to brace myself, then lean back, totally extend my right leg forward, lift the left leg slightly to unlock it, swivel on the right heel, and plop down on the seat—a clunky, noisy procedure that didn't ever get any more finessed with practice. It was not dainty.

"We can't do this!" I whisper-shrieked.

"What do you mean, *we*? I can't get in there," Dave said.

"I can't sit down, let alone stand up. What are we going to do?" The *we* question again.

"Here, just put your feet straight out and I'll lower you down."

"Wait! I've gotta pull my pants down!" I said. The plane lurched, pitching me into Dave's chest. "Don't move," I said. I leaned against him and buried my head in his armpit. As I fumbled with the button on my jeans, the only thing that kept me from falling was the wall Dave's body created. There was no way I could hold on to anything and pull my pants down at the same time. *Next time we do this*, I told myself, *I'm going to wear underpants with a quick-release crotch*. I started to laugh as I imagined rolling through the aisles at Victoria's Secret. I was out of breath when I finally got my pants down.

Dave began to lower me, but I stopped him. "We can't do this. It's too small for both of us. The door won't close."

I felt a bead of sweat slide down my neck and spine. I hated the fact that I'd just used the word *can't* several times in the past two minutes. The word I had sworn not to use while still in the hospital in Salzburg. Instead, I tried to say things like "This is hard" and "Isn't there another way?"

"Well, it's already done," he said, stepping back and bracing himself in the doorframe as the plane swayed slightly to one side.

The bathroom door stayed open. With his slender body, Dave blocked as best he could what now looked to me to be a ginormous doorway. My face burned and my bladder clenched. I dropped my shoulders and closed my eyes in an attempt to force my body to relax. *Traveling used to be fun. Now it's mortifying*. Dave stood there as if this were an everyday occurrence. *How does he do that? Like this is no big deal, like this is something people see every day.*

I thought back to the beach and the many other occasions when Dave had acted as if nothing bad had ever happened to us, as if we were the same as we'd been a year ago. *Well, I guess, if he can do it, I can do it*, I thought. *Maybe the gawkers think they're watching the newest members of the mile-high club. Yeah, I kinda like that thought.* I liked that idea, but, of course, it wasn't true.

Back in our seats, I sat pensively. The giggles and enthusiasm were gone. My spontaneity had been squelched. I leaned back and pretended to float weightless over a beautiful, grassy field with lemon-yellow crocuses, clumps of cotton-ball sheep, and neatly stacked wood. My winged arms and rudder legs propelled me over a rushing river, whooshing up through gossamer clouds, banking right and swooping over craggy, snow-crested mountains. I was invincible.

An announcement, first in German, then in English, interrupted my fantasy: "Good morning, ladies and gentlemen. We are starting our descent into the Rhein-Main Airport in Frankfurt, Germany. Please return to your seats for the remainder of the flight. Local time is 8:45 a.m. Flight attendants, prepare for landing." Dave and I prepared ourselves.

As we descended the stairs onto the tarmac, cold, fresh air greeted us. When we entered the terminal, Dave was on the lookout for the luggage carousels, I for the women's restroom.

"Hey," I said as soon as I spied the DAMENTOILETTE sign. "Let's stop there first."

Dave set our carry-on bags on the immaculate tile floor and stretched his body side to side. It had been more than twenty-four hours since his last run, but he looked relaxed. I walked with my quad cane, toy soldier–style, into a vast, modern-looking bathroom with what must have had twenty to thirty roomy stalls. I took the first vacant one and sighed as I locked the door and sat down on the toilet. But my relief was short lived.

When I put my foot out in front of me, turned, and looked for something to put my hand on so I could push and lever myself up, there was nothing. Grab bars would have been nice but hadn't come into vogue yet. Most, if not all, toilets in the United States at that time had the water tank mounted securely behind the seat, either in the wall or in the floor. I'd practiced this maneuver incessantly while learning to walk at the naval hospital. After perfecting it, I'd gained my freedom to be away from the house for extended periods of time.

I looked around and felt a twinge of anxiety. *There has to be a water tank somewhere!* And then I saw it—high up on the wall above my head. I was in trouble. Not sure what to do, I turned slightly, put my hand on the back of the toilet seat, and tried to push up. I was able to prop my body up and fully extend my strong arm, locking my elbow, but all that did was lift me a few inches. I repositioned myself and tried again. And again. *No way that will work.* I sat still and looked for another solution. I saw none.

And then I looked at the locked door. If I could open it, perhaps some compassionate fellow traveler could help me. That would be no more humiliating than the show I'd given my fellow plane passengers just hours before.

I grabbed my cane and tried to push the lock open, but it was too far away. My heart raced; my hands and upper lip began to sweat. I started to panic. I'd been there for a long time now. I was pretty sure Dave was pacing outside, wondering if I was okay. I looked at the space under the door and considered sliding off the toilet and onto the floor. Running out of ideas, I realized that I needed to get Dave to help me. I took a deep breath.

"I need help!"

Nothing happened.

A little louder. "Help! Does anyone speak English?"

Another wait.

"Can. Anyone. Speak. English?"

And then a "Yes, I speak English. What do you need?" floated toward me. "Where are you?"

"Over here. I can't get out."

The voice moved toward me and stopped on the other side of the locked door.

"My husband's name is Dave. He's waiting outside for me. Can you find him and get him to come in and help me?"

"Yes, but I think I will need to clear the bathroom first," the bodiless voice said.

She spoke loudly in German and then English to get everyone's attention: "A lady in here needs help, and we need to have her husband come in to help her."

The bodiless voice moved away from me, but I heard it projecting toward the entrance. "Dave . . . Is there anyone here named Dave?"

I heard Dave's faint but concerned response. "Yes. I'm Dave."

"Your wife needs help." Behind her, what sounded like dozens of women walked out, chattering and telling those outside not to go in.

I sat and waited, mortified but also relieved as I heard Dave walking toward me, calling out, "Where are you?"

"Right here," I said.

"Can you unlock the door?"

"No."

"Okay," he said, from right outside the door.

I heard movement; then, suddenly, his grinning face was looking up at me as he slid on his back under the door.

"My knight in shining armor!" I said.

He reached up to unlock the door, stood, hauled me up, and wrapped me in a hug.

"It's okay," he said. "It'll be funny in a few years."

We walked out together, my arm gripping his. The throng of waiting women cheered.

Still feeling a little sheepish, we found an airport wheelchair for me to use and followed signs to the departure gates. Our connecting flight to Stuttgart was scheduled to leave in an hour, which left us plenty of time. Or so we thought.

We approached the podium and handed the gate attendant our tickets. He took one look at me and the wheelchair and flew into action.

"Please give me your ticket. And your passport, please," he said to me, first in German, then in heavily accented English when I looked puzzled.

"You must go. Now!"

I tugged on Dave's shirt. "This guy is telling me I need to go with him," I said. "And that I need my passport and ticket."

"*You* need to get your luggage and go through customs," the attendant said to Dave.

Dave barely glanced at me as he handed me my passport and ticket. He then turned back to the desk. "Where is customs?"

"Down that hall and out those doors," the attendant said with a nod.

As Dave stepped in the direction indicated, another airport employee pushed my wheelchair toward a nearby elevator. I twisted around and pointed back at Dave. "I'm traveling with him. I need to stay with him." He paid no attention to me. He was on a mission.

And then I was gone. Whisked into an elevator. Down to ground level. Out a double-locked basement door. Into the bright sunlight. On the tarmac again.

An airport ambulance arrived. Its back doors flew open, and a wheelchair ramp unfolded. I was pushed up into the ambulance. The doors slammed closed, and straps appeared out of nowhere to tie down the wheelchair. Off we went. I leaned over so I could see out the window. We wove between monstrous planes before emerging into a wide-open space. The attendant looked at my ticket again, said something to the driver in German, and we veered off to the right.

In no time, we were sitting under the belly of a large plane. People appeared seemingly from nowhere, and a lift was rolled over. My attendant and I were placed on it. And, just like that, I was aboard an empty airplane. Without Dave.

I stood up, took hold of my cane, and slowly walked sideways to my assigned seat. I felt vulnerable, a little like a kid again, wanting my mom or dad to rescue me.

The other passengers on our flight began to board. Dave wasn't among them. The other passengers found and settled into their seats. No Dave. The captain and flight attendants made their announcements and readied the aircraft for departure. Still no Dave. They closed the doors and buckled themselves into their jump seats. The engines revved; we thundered down the runway and lifted off. Without Dave.

I had no idea where he was as I hurtled off into the sky. I was suddenly and unexpectedly independent. With a burst of elation, I sat up straighter, loosened my seat belt, and smiled. I looked like everyone else. I was on my own, going somewhere, ready for adventure. Even though he wasn't in the seat next to me, Dave's support and hard work had put me there. We were together even when apart.

Four hours after mine, Dave's plane touched down. We were together again. Interdependent but not dependent on each other to go where we wanted to go.

~

A cuckoo clock sang its 9:00 a.m. song in Stuttgart, Germany. The merry, dirndled wooden girls laughed at me as my internal clock argued, insisting that it was really midnight.

"Your mom's dinners are even more exquisite than I remember," I said to Dave, hiding a yawn.

I hoped my second cup of strong black coffee would convince my tired body to buck up and fast-forward to morning.

The night before, Jack and Donna's apartment had been the scene of a dinner party—a reunion of sorts: a mix of the

Society for the Serendipitous Restoration of Social, Scientific, and Sexual Scintillation Among the Amorous, Erotic, and Occasionally Erratic Emmigrants [*sic*] and a few of Jack and Donna's current friends and neighbors. It was a poignant but celebratory event, with many hugs and kisses, champagne toasts, and an occasional happy tear.

"Should we warm up the leftover filet mignon and *pommes Anna?*" I asked Dave.

"No way. I don't think my body could handle it. How about toast, and maybe we split an apple or something?"

While I buttered the toast, Dave thumbed through his dad's stack of vinyl record jackets and stopped on one that made his face light up.

"How about this?" he said, flipping the cover in my direction. A joyous Julie Andrews, her arms flung wide open, seemed to jump from the sleeve and dance toward me out of an Austrian meadow. Dave slipped the disc from its paper sheath and carefully set the needle arm on the outer edge of the record. The faint chirping of a bird, crescendoing strings with a flute trill, and deepening horns announced the prelude, and then Julie Andrews serenaded us.

The hills weren't the only thing alive with the sound of music.

"Here's to vacation," I said as I raised my coffee mug.

Three days before, Dave had finished his oral boards in therapeutic radiology at the Executive West Hotel in Louisville, Kentucky, an event every radiology resident spends four years dreading and thousands of hours preparing for. I knew he was exhausted but at the same time elated to be back in Germany, getting ready to finish the vacation that had been so rudely interrupted the year before. He looked up from the *International Herald Tribune*, his head swaying as he mimed

Julie Andrews's "favorite things" line with a broad smile on his face.

"You know," I said, "you're one of my favorite things."

"And that's why I never feel sad," he said.

Dave was twenty-eight and I was thirty years old, but *The Sound of Music* still sent chills up our spines. His parents were at work, and we had no plans. After clearing the table, I settled in on the couch with travel guides and maps and train schedules. I turned away from Dave's line of sight and surreptitiously unbuttoned the top of my shirt.

"So, which train should we try to catch to Salzburg tomorrow?" I asked, scooting over to make space for him on the couch.

"I think it's about a four-hour trip, so we don't need to go very early," he replied.

"Come over here and show me," I said in a husky voice. I sweetened the proposition with a little cleavage reveal and boob jiggle.

He casually but eagerly came closer.

"Show you, huh? Show you what?" he whispered in my ear as he snuggled up next to me. I slid my hand up his leg and leaned back invitingly. We'd learned to go slowly and gently when I had my fake legs on, because the tops of the hard fiberglass sockets put Dave's manhood at imminent risk—a level of excitement in lovemaking that wasn't necessarily a good thing.

As if in benediction, symphonic strings, then harp and chorus, joined in, swelling to a mighty climax: mountains, streams, rainbows, dreams.

～

The next day, I held Dave's arm tightly as we walked into the Unfallkrankenhaus. It had been nine months since I'd arrived near death in an ambulance. When we passed the front desk of the trauma hospital, someone recognized us and shouted,

"*Die Amerikaner sind wieder da*," sending out the joyous news that we were back and that I was walking. I wasn't on a litter, fighting for life. I had legs. Whole. Standing up and walking again. Doctors, nurses, orderlies, and other staff soon joined us in the lobby for a raucous and tearful reunion.

Later that week, as I followed Dave over a narrow Venetian canal on a rough cobblestone bridge, he turned around and snapped, "Come on, what is taking you so long?" Stunned, I stopped. I stared daggers at him before we burst out laughing. We were walking. We were traveling for five days without a wheelchair. Just like every other young couple. *We might look a little funny, and we certainly are slow, but we're doing it!* Fake legs, real legs—it didn't matter.

Within days, Dave was sneaking sidewise glances at me. "Your skin looks good. Glowing, even," he said with a sly grin.

Then more to the point, a few days later: "You look pregnant. What do you think?"

I'd forgotten that Dave adores pregnant women. To him, they're sexy, vibrant, and alluringly beautiful. *Uh-oh. Now I'm in trouble. He won't be able to keep his hands off me.*

In a sudden rush, my cheeks felt hot. *How can he tell?* His green eyes twinkled. His mustached grin spread to his ears, and he gently wrapped his arms around me. My stomach lurched as I turned away. I tried to smile as the room closed in on me. *This can't be. But maybe it is. Maybe this explains why my breasts have been feeling warm and swollen for the past few days.* I looked up at Dave again. His eyes were brimming with tears. Then he hugged me so hard that I couldn't breathe. This was a leap forward in our lives as a couple, cementing our bond even more firmly and moving us one step closer to normal.

"You might want to sit down," I said to my mother one afternoon
near the end of my first trimester. "I've got some good news."

"Oh?"

"Dave and I are going to have a baby."

Silence. And more silence. A really long silence.

"Oh, no! You can't be! How are you going to take care
of it?" she finally blurted out.

It was my turn to be speechless.

"Well, I think we'll be able to figure out how to do it.
Don't you want to be a grandmother?"

My mom and I had always had a great relationship, and
we talked easily to each other. Her questions and implied crit-
icism puzzled me.

She turned her head away and gazed out the window
awhile, before looking back into my eyes. After another pause,
she asked, "What will you do if Dave leaves you?"

There it was again: the gut-wrenching specter of the possibility that Dave might give up at some point and abandon
me. That I'd be unattractive, or too much work, or too boring
for him to want to stick around.

I gulped and forced a tiny smile. "I can't know for sure,
but I don't think he'll leave me. He really wants to have children—*our* children. Children who might turn out to be like
us. We think we can do it."

Suddenly, that beautiful, sweeping melody welled up inside
me, the song that has become a recurring theme and inspiration
for us: "A dream that will need all the love you can give."

~

I tried not to think about it, but when I did, the prospect of having
children scared me to death. I was all questions, few answers:

How will I feed them?

Can I change their diapers with one hand?

I can't push them in a stroller, put them in a car seat, or hold their hand and walk in the park.

What if something dangerous happens to them and I'm unable to save them?

And, finally: How will they feel as they grow older and realize how severely disabled their mom is? Will they think we've been selfish and given no thought to how weird their mother is and how my disability will embarrass them and limit their ability to live a fun, normal life?

On a positive note, I rationalized that the slow weight gain of pregnancy would help me strengthen my back and hip muscles—my new favorite muscles, the ones I used for my toy-soldier walk. Plus, it would be a huge distraction that would keep me from focusing on myself and make me learn how to do things quickly before we became a threesome. There was no good reason to keep putting it off. At thirty-one years of age, I would already be an old mom when the baby was born, eight years older than the average first-time mother in 1981.

When insecurity and abject fear threatened to overtake me, I forced myself to remember what Dave had said to me: "There's no difference between being disabled and being a dinosaur."

If T. rexes, with their itty-bitty arms, and triceratops, with no arms at all, could be moms, why couldn't I?

CHAPTER 6:

Independence Day

....

"Dave, I'm ready," I said, a little too sharply. It was the 6:30 a.m. ritual, and I detested it. I'd powdered my stumps, pulled the pantyhose on them, strapped on my fake legs and was squirming in my wheelchair. It was spring 1980, and we were living by ourselves in Dave's parents' house in San Diego.

"There's gotta be a way for me to put these on by myself," I grumbled as he knelt on the floor. I levered up and grabbed the edge of the dresser to steady myself. Dave, on the other hand, grinned lasciviously as he scooted in between my legs and looked up my crotch while he wrapped the loose end of a nylon around his wrist and pulled down to snug my leg into the socket of my prosthesis.

"Ooh, I like your panties," he said. "Especially these black ones."

I rolled my eyes and wished he'd hurry up.

"Hon, you've got the cutest ass. This is my favorite time of day."

"Well, I *hate* it. I *hate* being dependent, and I *hate* having you work so hard all the time." My voice choked and I gritted my teeth, trying not to turn this into a bitch session.

"Well, I *love* your black panties, and you turn me on." We had some variation of this conversation every morning, always initiated by Dave and always ending with a hug and a kiss when my legs were finally on. I smiled in spite of myself.

Dave rolled out of bed at four thirty every morning and pulled on an old T-shirt and shorts so he could get in a seven-mile run before six o'clock. Then Mr. Sweaty Body would haul me out of bed and plop me down on the floor of the shower, and we'd giggle a lot while lathering up—my turn to sit between his legs. There was no time for dilly-dallying, though, because every minute was scripted so we could eat breakfast, get my legs on, and get out the door. Dave dropped me off at the VA hospital or UCSD Medical Center, Hillcrest, and then drove downtown to the Naval Regional Medical Center in Balboa Park.

Eternal dependency was one of my earliest fears in the first days after the accident. Being incapable of going to the bathroom by myself, clumsily trying to eat, unable to move without assistance. Powerless, impotent, incapable, inept, inadequate, weak, unfit. Helpless. These words had never been in my vocabulary. Now they haunted me.

"Well, you know I can't go back to LA if I can't get these things on by myself." *There. It's out in the open.* I wanted to be able to live on my own again. I wanted Dave to be on his own again. And what if the worst happened? *What if Dave decides he's had enough and leaves me?* I wondered.

"I've got some ideas about something I can make that might work." One more tug on the last nylon; then he shoved the end of the nylon into the socket and screwed in the valve. "Something you can lean on and that will support you if you lose your balance; something to take my place. Sit down, and I'll show you what I've drawn."

Something to take his place. I hoped that would never happen, but I guessed it'd be good to be prepared.

The sketch was not much more than a scribble, but it looked brilliant. A three-by-three-foot piece of plywood on the floor with four vertical metal pipes, one attached at each corner. Horizontal bars would attach the tops of the pipes to each other, leaving one side open, like a square with one side missing.

"You can push your wheelchair up to the open side and lock it in place. Once you've pulled the pantyhose up on your residual limbs, you'll reach for your prostheses, pull them to you, and slide them onto your stumps. Then you'll buckle the straps around your pelvis and waist and stand up. Once you're upright, you can lean over, with the back bar supporting your waist, reach down and grab the ends of the nylons, and pull yourself the rest of the way into your prostheses." He paused for a moment to take a breath. "After you tuck in the ends of the nylons, you can screw in the valves, push yourself upright, pull up your jeans, and voilà—you'll be whole again!"

I laughed out loud at the cartoon in my mind. The upper half of a person rolls in to meet up with a lower-half person. A few grunts and groans later, the torso can ambulate and the legs can vocalize.

"If you stand up, I'll measure you so I'll know how tall to make Iron Mike."

"Iron who?"

"Iron Mike. Your new best friend," Dave replied.

Hmmm . . . a ménage à trois? Why not!

Grasping the left armrest of my wheelchair and pivoting on my right heel, I strong-armed myself forward, hoping like hell that I wouldn't push so hard that I toppled over and smashed my face.

"See," Dave said, "Iron Mike will keep you safe when I'm not around. If you push too hard getting up, he'll catch you with his strong metal arms so you can't fall."

Dave's sketch became a reality. A week and sixty-five bucks later, the three black arms and four black legs came to life in the family room. That night, I unstrapped my legs and propped them in Iron Mike's embrace; they reposed there while Dave carried me upstairs, where the rest of us slumbered. One more step on my road to independence.

By midspring, I walked well enough that Dave started taking me to the VA hospital to spend the day in the radiology department where I sat in on readouts and conferences. It was the easiest way to build my strength and learn how to maneuver without the responsibility or pressure of reading films. For a few minutes a day, I felt a flash of my old self when I made the correct diagnosis on an X-ray image.

For the first few months, all I thought about was walking. No, actually, what I really thought about was falling. My toy-soldier gait is unique, and in case people didn't see me, they'd definitely hear my *thump, thud, thump, thud* cadence as I made my way slowly down the halls. Even though I'm a small person, I take up a lot of space as I walk with my wide-base stride, by placing my cane out in front of me and to the left to protect the space around me. My biggest fear was that I'd be knocked down, so I hugged the right side of hallways, hoping the wall would break my fall if I lost my balance. Imagine walking on stilts with knees.

I thought back to the first lists I wrote with my left hand the week after the accident. We were making good progress, but the clock was still ticking on one thing: finishing my residency. My yearlong medical leave of absence would be complete at the end of August, so I had to be back to work by September 1980 to fulfill the last nine months of my residency. If I was even a week or two short of training, I'd have to wait another whole year to take the exam—an unacceptable option.

Dave and I had been in complete agreement about the importance of my becoming a radiologist. I'd spent many hours during the weeks in Salzburg dreaming and planning my return to finish my residency. In my bleakest hours, I found hope by imagining myself at a radiology viewbox—dictating films, calling clinicians with results, joking with my colleagues. All of this typically happens in a darkened room—a room in which people wouldn't see my missing legs and arm, a room in which my radiologic interpretations would help my fellow doctors save lives and my empathy and humor would brighten the day.

When I had my doctor hat on, it was easy to forget my funny walk and missing arm. I felt worthwhile and needed.

"Do you think you can find a roommate? Would your sister live with you again?" Dave was washing the dinner dishes. It had been a month since our return from Europe, and both of us were tired. A fork slipped out of my hand and clattered to the floor.

"I love my sister but I don't want a roommate."

"I know, but you're pregnant. This is my baby, too, and I can't help you when I'm one hundred and ten miles away. What if you fall? How are you going to get help? How will you get to the phone?" His voice kept getting louder.

I froze, unable to respond. I was going to LA no matter what. Dave's temper and my passivity or aversion to confrontation are an issue between us. He can "see red" instantly. It takes me forever to get mad. But watch out—if you push me enough, I won't talk to you for three days. "You ass-holy shithead" is my favorite term of endearment for him when I've reached that stage.

I took a deep breath and waited. I was concerned about *him*. I suspected that this accident and recovery were easier for me because I could take physical control and work hard to make things better. The more I sweated, the stronger I got.

While Dave obviously did most of the grunt work, he had more mental uncertainty. *Am I physically strong enough to do what the doctors have said is not possible? Will I persevere? Will I get depressed?* He also had more anger about the accident than I did. And then financial security was a huge issue. It was going to cost a lot of money to modify or build a house, to adapt a car for me to drive, to pay for household help. And finally, who would take care of me if he couldn't, and what would it cost?

I was convinced that his addiction to running was probably what would save him. To him, a day without running is worse than a day without food. It's where he sorts through a myriad of issues, airs them out in his mind, creates solutions, and packs them back into his brain so he can deal with them as the day wears on. I learned only recently how he felt and what he did on those early morning runs the year after the accident.

The radiology department at UCSD had offered to let me finish my residency there, but I'd declined. It would take a while for me to learn how to operate the equipment with one hand. I'd be unable to perform angiograms, bronchograms, lymphangiograms, myelograms, and some of the less invasive procedures. I was sure I'd be slow at first and might not be able to pull my weight. It seemed better that I return to the White Memorial Medical Center where everyone knew me as a hardworking, gung-ho resident and would be cheering me on. My dad worked at the same hospital, and my parents lived about twenty minutes away, so they could help me if need be. Plus, who could know how my pregnancy would go? But the overarching reason I wanted to go back was so I could live on my own again.

Am I being selfish and self-centered? Am I pushing an even bigger burden of worry onto Dave? I knew that he wanted to take care of but not smother me. He still wanted me to be a doctor but worried that the collision of studying for boards, figuring out how to live by myself, and carrying our baby was an invitation for failure or discouragement or depression. He knew I was strong, but we'd been told that it takes a bilateral above-the-knee amputee four times the amount of energy to walk as it takes a normal person. Add to that the energy that pours from a woman's body into her baby while it grows, and cap that off with the necessity of studying for boards at least two hours every night after getting home from a full day at work.

After things settled down a bit, I looked at Dave and said, "I've made a timetable for myself to start studying." I handed him an outline of the books I needed to digest in the next twelve months. Lists are our way of tackling problems, and beginning to study would get me revved up for moving back to LA. "If I get started now, I think I'll have time to review the teaching file at least one last time just before the exam."

"Sounds reasonable to me," he said. "While you've been doing that, I've been thinking about making it easier for you to climb the stairs here at home." Now, that was big. In the beginning, staircases might as well have been Mount Everest, so I'd put a lot of effort into mastering them.

Difficulty going up and down stairs had been very problematic for me. Everything I needed always seemed to be above or below where I was. This dramatized one of my major shortcomings: disorganization. Dave is constantly annoyed by my "shit piles." He, on the other hand, is a neatnik who knows where everything is in his life. I'm the one always looking for things, wondering where I left them. *It is so like him to be constantly devising ways to make my life closer to normal. I'm going to have to start paying attention to things. I can't make his life miserable by picking up after me.*

"How big is this new man?" I asked, laughing.

"Well, I couldn't find anyone as strong and good-looking as I am, so I've settled on having a handrail installed on the left-side wall going up the stairs."

The railing was installed about a week later, and we moved Iron Mike up into our room the same day.

"Okey-dokey, here I go." I wedged my forearm between the wall and handrail, grabbing it tightly. Taking a deep breath, I hiked my right hip up and threw my leg up, levering myself onto the first step. Leaning right, I dragged my left leg up . . . and then I was standing eight inches closer to our bedroom. At this rate, I'd have to start getting ready for bed ten minutes before Dave every night.

The next morning, I stood at the top of the stairs, wobbling a little on the deep, yellow shag carpet. The fastest way would be to butt-slide down, but I didn't think Dave would be too impressed with that. So I turned around, clutched the railing, leaned over, and, putting my left foot down behind me, proceeded with my drunken-sailor, backward trek downstairs. Each step brought me more independence.

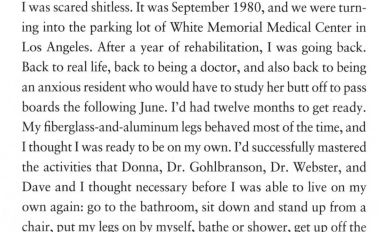

I was scared shitless. It was September 1980, and we were turning into the parking lot of White Memorial Medical Center in Los Angeles. After a year of rehabilitation, I was going back. Back to real life, back to being a doctor, and also back to being an anxious resident who would have to study her butt off to pass boards the following June. I'd had twelve months to get ready. My fiberglass-and-aluminum legs behaved most of the time, and I thought I was ready to be on my own. I'd successfully mastered the activities that Donna, Dr. Gohlbranson, Dr. Webster, and Dave and I thought necessary before I was able to live on my own again: go to the bathroom, sit down and stand up from a chair, put my legs on by myself, bathe or shower, get up off the floor if I fell, go up and down stairs, and walk long distances comfortably with a cane. It had been hard work—sweaty, grueling, and oftentimes discouraging—but I'd done it. *We'd* done it.

My priority when I got back to work was to identify bathrooms in the radiology department that would suit my needs. *Wonder if they'll let me put up a LINDA'S BATHROOM sign.* Likewise, I was choosy about which chairs I sat in. While sturdy chairs with armrests are my preference, I've tamed chairs on wheels—as found in most offices—by backing them up to a wall or desk so they can't roll away from me when I fully extend my right leg, throw myself up with my muscled left arm, pivot around on my right heel while swinging my left leg out into extension, and stand up straight without teetering too much. There are two risks to this maneuver: the chair could tip over or roll away while I land on my behind, or I could use too much force when I thrust myself upright, and then topple over, flat on my face.

I never practiced falling because of the risk that I might break my only remaining extremity, but I mentally prepared for this possibility by telling myself that if I thought it was going to happen, I'd pull my arm in close to my body and tuck and roll, kind of like what big, burly football dudes do every Sunday on national television. I hoped I'd never have to do it.

Setting aside the concerns about living on my own, I knew my primary challenge was to get into a routine of studying for the American Board of Radiology exam. It was a half-day oral exam in Louisville, Kentucky. The first part of board certification was a written exam that I'd passed a few weeks before the accident. Over the next ten months, I'd need to look at thousands of images and read the major texts about seven topics that were on the exam then: musculoskeletal, central nervous system, pediatric, gastrointestinal/genitourinary, thoracic, cardiovascular, and nuclear medicine. I was just like every other radiology resident in the country, trying to balance work with study. But I also knew that I *had* to pass, because, as a disabled female, I'd never get a job if I didn't pass the first time around.

And I wanted Dave to be proud of me.

In addition, I needed to figure out how to operate the machines, start IVs, and dictate and interpret films in a timely fashion. I played all the scenes in my mind and had a backup plan for every scenario. Oh, and then there was the fact that I was pregnant.

I was moving back into the high-rise apartment building, located behind White Memorial Medical Center, where I'd lived for the three years preceding the accident. I sat quietly for a few moments, recalling the first time I'd moved into this building—one week after graduating from medical school. My boyfriend, Dave, and I had rented a U-Haul truck in Redlands and gleefully packed my furniture and clothes for the one-hour drive out Interstate 10 to East LA.

He had worked for Mayflower during college summers and knew how to do this. The dishes were packed carefully in paper and stacked in dish boxes; my clothes hung in wardrobe boxes. He'd loaded my furniture, miscellaneous boxes, skis, and all my camping equipment onto the van in military order. My pride and joy had been a classic, mint-green Bianchi racing bike with sew-up tires that made me feel like a superathlete when I sped along country roads in San Timoteo Canyon or up into the San Bernardino Mountains to Oak Glen. There were clothes for every occasion, hiking boots, and shoes. Lots of shoes. Imelda Marcos would have been envious.

We'd giggled and flirted with each other. Deep down, we had a lot of uncertainties. Would our relationship survive the next four years, 110 miles apart? Had we chosen the right specialties? For me, the scariest thing was that, two days later, I'd put on a stiffly starched, new white coat with my name stitched on it: Linda K. Olson, MD. It seemed to me that seven days was not enough to turn a fourth-year medical student into a doctor, but that's what happens. It was scary to think about seeing patients on my own, writing orders in the middle of the night, waiting for my pager to go off, and possibly not knowing what to do.

I'd been scared and excited then, too, but this time I had a ground-floor apartment that had been graciously modified for my use. Within the first few months after my accident, the administration at White Memorial Medical Center informed us of its unanimous decision to create a wheelchair-accessible apartment for me so I could return and finish my residency. This was a full ten years before the passage of the Americans with Disabilities Act.

As we pulled into the parking lot, I saw my new place and grinned. Dave, my boyfriend turned husband, was grinning and crying at the same time. It was bittersweet to see the newly painted, blue handicapped parking space welcoming us to a ground-floor apartment—a space I wouldn't be able to use, because I couldn't drive. It wasn't clear to either of us if I'd ever be able to drive. Several times I'd sat in the driver's seat of our car, experimenting with different ideas, like strapping my fake feet to the gas and brake so I'd accelerate and stop, or getting an artificial arm with a hook on it that could attach to a ring on the steering wheel for turning. I always came back to the fact that I'd need two extremities to drive: one for gas/brake and another for steering. My one remaining extremity was strong and worked really well, but it wasn't extraordinary enough to perform this miracle. I kept pushing down the fear that I'd never be able to drive. *I will do anything. It must happen. It will happen. For the time being, I can look out the window and imagine Dave parking his puke-green Toyota Corona there when he comes to spend weekends with me.*

A short sidewalk led directly from the parking spot to a sliding glass door that had been modified to become the entry, which I accessed with a remote-controlled, battery-operated garage-door opener. With the click of a button, the door slid open and I could walk or roll in. Click the button again, and the door closed and locked. Pretty cool! A remodel of the bathroom provided me with a wheelchair-accessible shower, sink, and toilet, plus grab bars on three walls.

We brought very little with us. Furniture gets in the way of my wheelchair. A dining room table and two chairs, a small TV, a few kitchen appliances, and, of course, Iron Mike. Dave hauled the mattress and box spring into the bedroom and left it on the floor without a frame. This functioned as a safety backup. If I fell, I could butt-walk across the floor, pull myself up onto the bed, and stand up if I had my legs on or get into my wheelchair if I didn't have my legs on. I had just a few clothes—baggy pants and formless dresses that I could grow into as my pregnancy progressed—and only one pair of shoes, which stayed on my fake feet twenty-four hours a day.

I'd had my first, temporary set of legs for ten months. Permanent legs are not made until the soft tissues of the residual limb have stopped shrinking, usually three to six months after amputation. But because I was pregnant, things would continue to change for several more months. My doctors decided that it would be best if I waited until after the baby was born for my permanent, suction-socket legs to be made.

Every morning, I pushed myself to the open side of Iron Mike and locked my wheelchair in place. Every morning, I had to look down at my stubby, scarred, and puckered legs that extended only about eight inches in front of me, leaving a lot of empty space in my wheelchair. Pulling a pair of pantyhose up to my waist, I smoothed them over my residual legs and gazed at the twenty to thirty inches of empty, wrinkled nylon that dangled over the edge of the seat. Still seated, I took each artificial leg from its resting place and pulled it partway on what was left of my real legs, threading the nylon pantyhose out through the hole at the front lower end of each

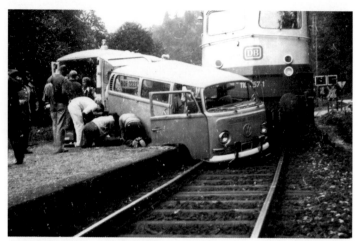

Paramedics leaning over me on the ground next to the van. August 27, 1979.
Photo © Bavarian State Police Berchtesgaden

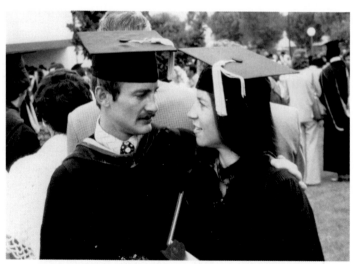

One of the happiest days of my life, graduating with Dave from
medical school at Loma Linda University, Class of 1976-A.
Photo © Albert L. Olson

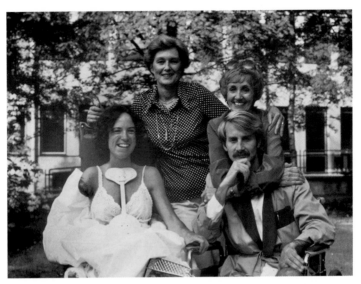

*Adrian (top left) and Donna (top right) hugging Dave and me
a few days after the accident. Afternoons in the hospital garden
were excellent therapy, maybe because of the Austrian beers
we bought in the hotel lobby? Photo © Jack Hodgens*

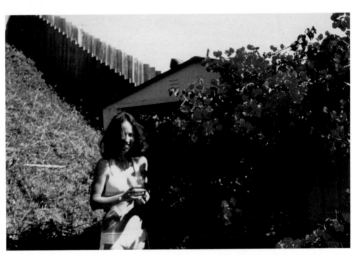

*I endeared myself to my future in-laws by weeding in their backyard.
I endeared myself to Dave by wearing a bikini when weeding.
Photo © David Hodgens*

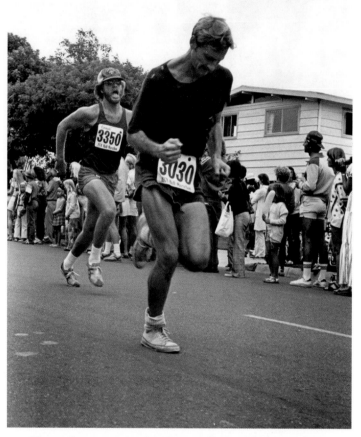

Vintage Dave running in his "Connie All-stars" (Converse All-Star shoes), baggy socks, ratty tee shirt with stretched out neck, and the dogged determination that has carried him more than 80,000 miles since we've known each other. Photo © Sports Photos, Coronado, CA

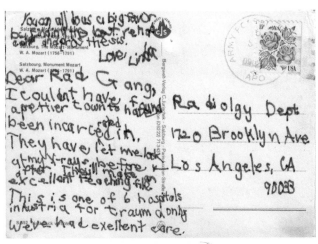

Reconnecting with my radiology colleagues, "Rad Gang," at the White Memorial Medical Center six days after the accident. It was hard to spell correctly as I started writing with my left hand. Photo © Linda Olson

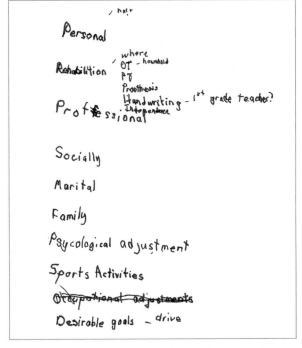

This is the list of priorities we made the first week. Dave made me record it so I could practice writing with my left hand. Photo © Linda Olson

<u>FROM:</u>

The Society for the Serendipitous Restoration of
Social, Scientific and Sexual Scintillation
Among the Amourous, Erotic and Occasionally
Erratic Emmigrants to the Bavarian Barracks
in Bertchesgaden

<u>To:</u>

The Famously Fantastic, Fabulously
Realistically and Resolutely Responsive Regenerates
Confined In a Cozy Korner of the Krankenhaus

<u>Greetings:</u>

Having duly considered cautiously the
characters of the confinee in question with
the definite difficulties that developed undoing
(temporarilly) the dosings of the most durable
dose in the domain of diabolical diagnostic
designees, the Society awards the meticulous
marks in management measures initiated by
the ingenuous ingenue and her consent in
commodiously comfortable Krankenhaus
cohabitation.

Bertchesgaden University for

Mature Students

" Bums "

The very lengthy and alliterative introduction to the "Report Card"
created in the evenings by our families and friends after they'd
had dinner . . . and perhaps a drink or two. Photo © Linda Olson

REPORT of PROGRESS

Achiever	O	(K) ~~xxxx~~ knowledgable	O
Borborygmi	E	Odoferous	F
Cursive Writing	S+	Passionate	OH! oh!
Defecation	S-	Quiet	F
Exhibitionist	E	Resourceful	O
Flatulence	S	Sadonfamously sexual	O
"Dusty"	O	Temptress	OH+
Horny	OH!	Urination	S
Irrepressible	O	Virtuous	F+
Juvenile	S	Warm (Ich bin)	O
Kissable	O	X rated	O 'OH'
Lovable	O	You are Terrifi	!
Manner (bedside)	NA	Ze END	?

O = OUTSTANDING
E = EXCELLENT
S = SATISFACTORY
F = FAILING

Using the alphabet to grade our condition in the
hospital infused some crazy humor into everyone's lives
during those first three weeks. Photo © Linda Olson

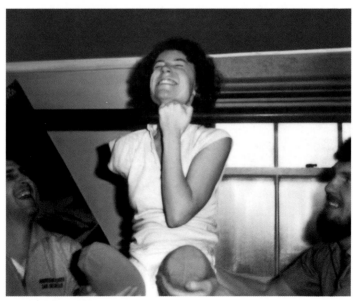

Learning how to do one-armed chin-ups in physical therapy with the help of
two Navy techs. We always made it look like fun. Photo © Donna Pavlick

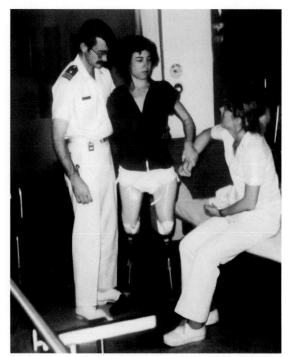

Dave and Donna Pavlick helping me stand in my first set of legs that looked like they'd come from a plumber's supply store. The rigid sockets were strapped around my pelvis and attached to metal knees and pipes which were affixed to feet with non-articulating ankles. They were just about as comfortable as it sounds. Photo credit unknown

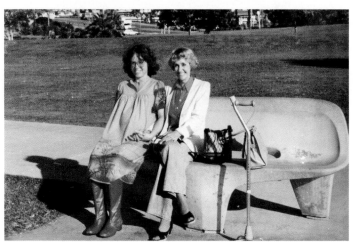

Resting after a walk with Donna at Mission Bay Park, the day before Tiffany was born. I kept those boots on my prostheses twenty-four hours a day–including during labor and delivery. Photo © Adrian Johnston

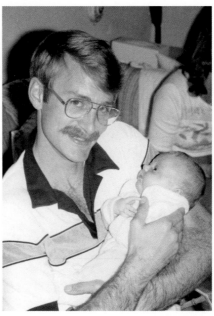

Dave holding Tiffany soon after she was born. Having children fulfilled a lifelong dream of his. Photo © Linda Olson

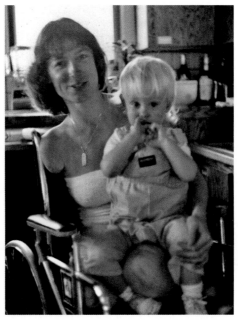

Linda and Tiffany. There was always at least one kid on my lap until they were three or four years old. Photo © David Hodgens

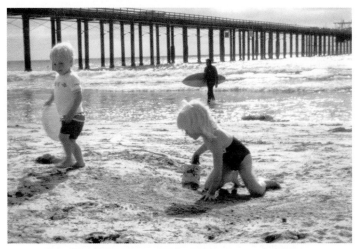

*The beach north of Scripps Pier is where Dave took me in my
bikini a couple of months after the accident and where we went
with the kids once or twice a week as they were growing up.
This was our home away from home. Photo © Linda Olson*

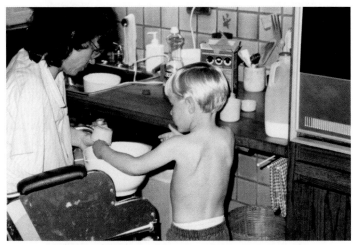

*Brian helping me cook. This is the part of the kitchen that we built at
wheelchair height. It was also perfect for children. Photo © David Hodgens*

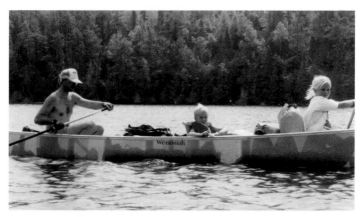

First camping trip to Yellowstone Lake when Brian was 5
and Tiffany was 8 years old. This began our tradition of annual
wilderness adventures with the Cox family. Photo © Linda Olson

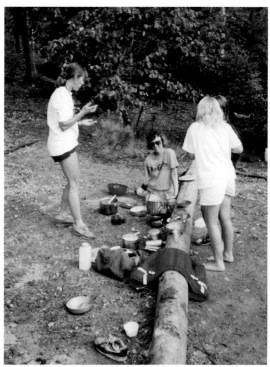

Carla, Heidi, Tiffany and I in our Yellowstone kitchen
where my very important job was to boil water and cook on
a tiny backpacking stove. And to ration the reward for
paddling all day—M&M's. Photo © David Hodgens

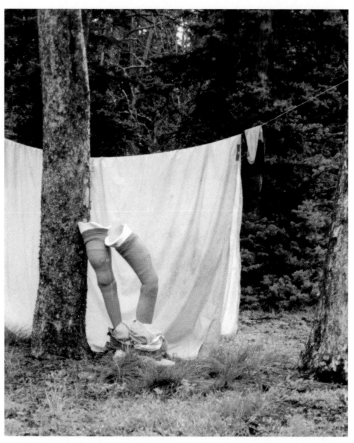

This serendipitous photo of my legs resting up against a tree in our camp in Yellowstone is one of my favorite pictures. It embodies my life after the accident; being able to adapt and get out and go with or without legs.
Photo © Linda Olson

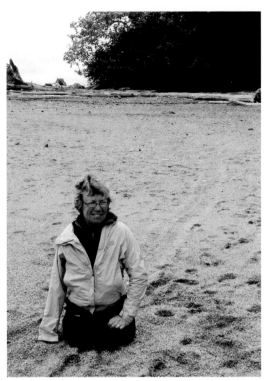

If you look carefully you can see my distinctive butt-walking tracks
behind me in the sand making it pretty easy to tell where I've been.
Photo © Trilby Cox

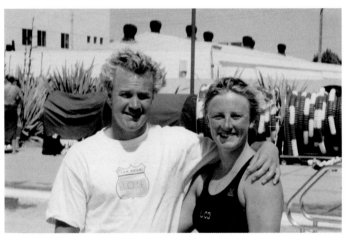

Brian and Tiffany grew up playing water polo at San Diego Shores with
Doug Peabody and went on to play varsity water polo at University of
California, Davis. This sport created a second family for them and helped
define their lives even past college. Photo © Linda Olson

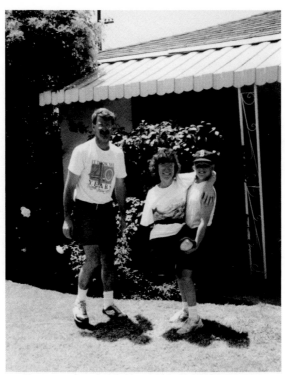

Tiffany was very proud of being able to carry me at age 11.
Photo © Albert L. Olson

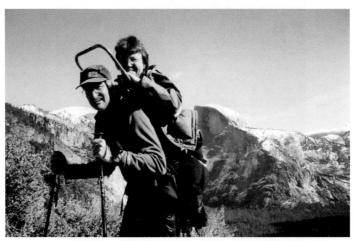

Dave has carried me many miles in backpacks like this that he modified
with a drop-down shelf for me to sit on. People coming toward us thought
he was a two-headed hiker. This was on the trail to Yosemite Falls
with Half Dome in the background. Photo by an unknown hiker

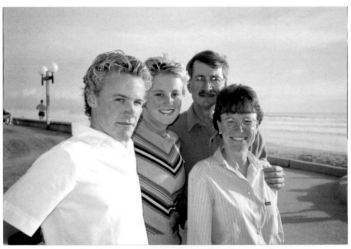

Thanksgiving at Coronado when Tiffany was in college and Brian in high school. Photo © Janice Hauser

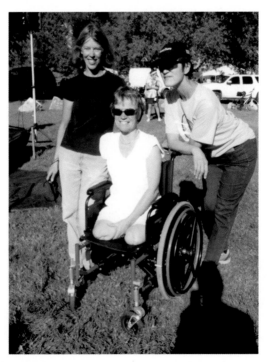

The middle-aged versions of me and my college roommates, Carla Wissner Cox and Juli Ling Miller. Along with their families, they've been the mainstays of our support team from the very beginning. Photo © David Hodgens

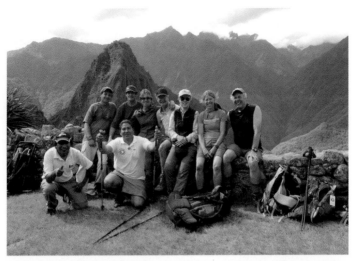

Yvonne Espinosa and Carla and Roger Cox accompanied us to Machu Picchu, one of the most amazing places we've been. Our guides, Edgar Mollinedo Quispe, Jose Ugarte de Souza, Benjamin Muniz Martinez, and Washington Gibaja Tapia carried me up and down the steep trails using the backpack Dave had made or pushing me in a wheelchair they'd made for me. Photo by an unknown hiker

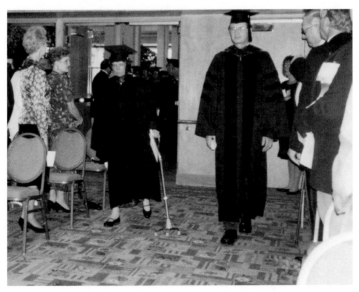

I was honored to become a Fellow of the American College of Radiology in 1993. This is one of the few pictures we have showing how I walked independently with a quad cane. Most people had no idea I was missing both my legs. Photo © David Hodgens

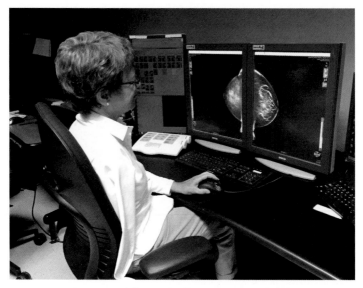

*I interpreted thousands of mammograms at UCSD
during my career. The perfect job for a one-arm radiologist.
Photo © Haydee Ojeda*

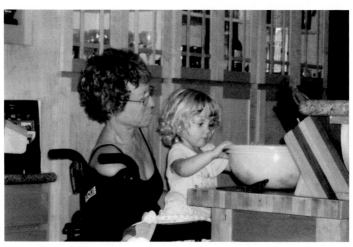

*Life has come full circle. Our granddaughter, Sierra, sitting in my
wheelchair and cooking with "No-Leg Grandma." Photo © David Hodgens*

socket, thereby tugging my legs partway into the sockets of the fake legs. I crisscrossed the wide, thick white straps over my pelvis and fastened them loosely. Taking a deep breath, I thrust myself upright and leaned over the front supporting rail, knowing that my wheelchair was right behind me if I fell. Grasping the protruding end of the nylon stocking at the end of the socket, I pulled steadily on the nylon so that it slid my thigh as deeply into the socket as possible. Then I stuffed the nylon back up into the small space left inside the end of the socket and screwed a valve into the hole. Left leg first, and then right leg. I stood up and wiggled my legs around to adjust the fit and tightness of the straps. Abracadabra—I was a biped again.

It was hard to believe, but it was real. *I'm going to be independent, living on my own again. And loving it! Who'd have thought that nylons, the bane of women's existence, would be my ticket to freedom?*

When we finished unpacking, Dave pushed me across the parking lot in my wheelchair, into the hospital, and down the hall to the back door of the radiology department. The big, automatic door-opener plate along the right side of the double doors meant one less obstacle in my world. I put on my happy face, ramped up my energy, pushed up out of my wheelchair, got my balance, and took hold of my quad cane. I took a deep breath and told myself to relax. *This is going to take all the willpower you have.*

As I walked down the long hallway, my perspective was very different. Walking required an enormous amount of energy but even more focus. I stayed near the right-side wall, pretending it would hold me up if I started to fall. My eyes were riveted to the linoleum, looking for slight irregularities so I wouldn't lose my balance and bash my face on the floor. I was so focused that it was impossible to talk and walk at the same time.

"Dr. Olson, is that you?" I heard astonishment in the heavily accented voice of the man who had been the radiology film file room director for many years.

I finished the step I was taking and planted my feet and quad cane firmly, in as stable a stance as I could muster, before I looked up. Dario was a small, shy, older Filipino man who walked quickly, in a hunched-over, self-effacing fashion. He got close to me and stopped, recognizing how precarious I looked standing in the middle of the hall. Tears trickled down his cheeks.

"We are sooo happy to see you back. Please tell me if I can help you." I let go of my cane and hugged him tightly.

I thump-thudded my way down the wide hallway, pausing at each room, thinking about the procedures we did in each one: sialograms, lymphangiograms, venograms, and hystero-salpingograms, upper GIs and barium enemas, bronchograms, and on and on. Radiologists perform all of these exams while standing in the room and insert catheters or needles for inject-ing contrast material so they can see an anatomical structure. We were just starting to do ultrasound studies. CT was not yet available at our hospital. Only two years earlier, in 1979, there were only two hundred CT scanners in the United States.

I was lucky to be near the end of my training. I already knew how to do all these procedures; now, I'd just learn how to do them in new ways. I thought I'd probably need to special-ize—that is, not be a general radiologist. But that was okay with me. I hated doing invasive procedures like angiograms anyway.

Dave and I stayed just long enough to say hi to everyone and confirm to ourselves that I could truly get around the whole department by myself. No more guessing. It was going to work.

Late that evening, balancing with my cane, I walked Dave out to his car as he readied to drive home to San Diego. Leaning against the car for support, I hugged him. We held each other tightly for a long time, tears running down our cheeks.

"Sorry I'm crying," I blubbered. "I'm really happy to be back. But it's a little scary. I don't want you to worry about me. I'm going to be just fine." I accidentally bumped my cane, and it fell over. I leaned down and grabbed it, steadying myself against the car door. "Remember when you moved me up here the first time? I was scared then, too." We were silent for a while. I remembered what it was like to stand there when I had feet that wiggled, bouncing from side to side with nervous energy. Feet that probably got cold standing there. Dave had supported me back then, just as he did again that night.

He hugged me even tighter. "Olsie, I *know* you can do it. And I know you *need* to do it. To be independent and finish your residency. You've worked really hard to get here tonight. I'm so proud of you."

"Thank you," I whispered, "for staying with me and helping me be strong. I don't think I could have done it without you."

He started the engine and switched on his headlights, watching to make sure my fake feet and cane got me safely back into my apartment. Then he was gone and I was on my own—again. We were regaining our independence. But it was different. We would be apart but closer than ever.

~

Dave and I resumed seeing each other only on weekends. Over the years, we've told our friends that it's one of the reasons we're still married—working hard during the week without each other and then playing together on the weekends. When I was on call, he drove up to see me. When I wasn't on call, I rode the Amtrak train from Union Station to Del Mar, just as I had for the three years before the accident. On Friday evenings, I loaded my wheelchair and overnight bag into a taxi that dropped me off at the train station, where I waited at the main entrance for an electric cart. I was just able to sidle up to it, pull myself semi-gracefully onto the seat, and settle in for a sedate ride through the ornate, high-ceilinged station, with its mission revival, art deco, and Spanish colonial architectural design. The floor and walls of the cool, cavernous hall were lined with travertine, terra cotta tiles, and inlaid marble strips. Enormous wrought-iron chandeliers floated high above the massive space. It's a recognizable setting that's appeared in many movies, and it welcomed me every week.

As soon as we crossed from the fancy floor to the concrete passageways, I had to hang on as the driver mashed the pedal to the floor and careened around corners, zooming up and down the subterranean ramps en route to the designated train track. I was usually the only passenger, and the driver knew I wouldn't complain about his speed-demon driving. Diesel-fuel fumes and the hiss and screech of nearby trains braking their way into the station assaulted my brain as the cart strained up the steep tunnel ramp and emerged onto the concrete platform.

Coasting to a stop at my train, I craned my neck, looking for my bevy of big black porters dressed in their navy-blue uniforms. They hovered over me as soon as I alighted from the cart, waiting to see if I needed help. The loud shushing, in-and-out breathing sound of the engine and wind blowing between the trains made walking with my cane an adventure. As I neared the huge metal wheels, I looked down between the edge of the concrete and train and saw the tracks and gravel rail bed.

I'd stared hard at the tracks the first few times I made this trek, challenging myself to see how I felt, to see if it would trigger any flashbacks or nightmares. Dave told me he did the same thing and had the exact same reaction—nothing.

We actually *like* riding trains. Being pragmatic people, we see them as a utilitarian means of transportation with multiple advantages over driving. No more traffic jams; easy to read or study for the two-and-a-half-hour trip or be lulled to sleep by the clickety-clacking tracks and gentle swaying rhythm of the car. And to feel refreshed at the other end, rather than angry, tired, nervous, or frazzled—what could be better?

"Hi, Doc, how ya doin'?" my favorite porter boomed. "It's my turn this week."

As soon as I got to the train steps, he leaned over and scooped me up in his big, strong arms while I crooked my left arm around his neck and broad shoulders. He swept me up the three or four steep steps into the train, whereupon he leaned over and gently lowered me inside the doorway. I left him with a hug, a thank-you, and a peck on the cheek. The porters all knew my story and appreciated that I had no fear of riding the trains with them every week. They knew I was pregnant and absolutely *loved* watching me glow and grow—being part of our family's journey. Dave says I have a way of making men happy by letting them carry me. None of these men seemed the least bit fazed by the fact that I'd gone from a lightweight to 110 pounds.

Upon arrival in Del Mar, I strained to see Dave, who was always either standing on the platform or walking alongside the train and peering into the windows as it slowed to a stop. When he saw me, he bounded up the steps and swept me down and out into his waiting car. The crash of the surf a couple of hundred yards away and the salty sea air were the prelude to another weekend together, enjoying each other and our impending new life.

I was elated to be back at work, where my days became predictable: be at morning conference by 7:00 a.m., work from eight to five, get supper in the hospital cafeteria, roll across the parking lot in my one-arm-drive manual wheelchair to my apartment, study for two hours, and go to bed. My pregnancy gave me more focus than I'd ever shown in my life. Scared I'd flunk my oral boards, I mapped out a rigid study schedule. I was even more scared that the baby would be too small or abnormal somehow, so I ate healthy food and got lots of rest.

The staff and my fellow residents enthusiastically reintegrated me into the program, figuring out ways for me to perform procedures and operate the radiologic equipment. But, most of all, they fluttered around me as if they were an army of surrogate parents, attending to the needs of my unborn child. Having me back at work while I had a new life within me was the icing on the cake. It helped all of us believe that things might get back to normal after all.

By the end of the first week, there was one elephant in the room. My fellow residents had been covering for me by starting IVs on my patients who needed intravenous contrast for procedures, but we all knew that had to change soon. It would have been nice if radiology technologists could have done it, but the state of California did not allow them to do so at the time.

"Hey, Linda."

I looked across the room to see Eric, one of my favorite techs, standing in the doorway. He held up a tourniquet and motioned me to follow him, which, like an idiot, I did. "Where are we going?" I asked when he turned left toward the hallway where all the radiologists' offices were.

"Dr. Sanders and Dr. Woesner want to see you."

Well, isn't that nice.

When I reached Dr. Sanders's office door, it seemed a little strange to see him sitting catty-corner at his desk, leaning over with his arm flat out in front of him. Dr. Sanders was a big man—six feet, five inches tall and weighing in at over two hundred pounds—who had a commanding presence and a booming, deep voice. I started to giggle when I saw him sprawled halfway across his huge mahogany desk, but the sight of Dr. Woesner pacing back and forth on the other side of the desk brought me back to my senses.

"You have to be able to start IVs, or you can't be a radiologist," Dr. Sanders said.

"I know, but I haven't figured out how to do it yet."

"Well, put your heart-shaped tush down in that chair and start by practicing on me."

I grasped the armrest of the chair, hoping it was sturdy enough to withstand my sit-down assault, and plopped down. As they hit the wood chair, my prostheses made a loud *clunk*, another of my new signature noises.

"Eric," Dr. Sanders said, "tie that tourniquet around my arm."

In no time, a big vein popped up, just waiting to be punctured with the butterfly needle that appeared out of thin air. Dr. Sanders had with his other hand already cleansed his arm with an alcohol swab and was waving his hand over it to air-dry the skin so it wouldn't sting when the needle entered it.

"I can't do this to you," I blurted out. "What if I miss?"

"And just who do you think is going to let you do this, other than me?" he demanded.

I'd worked there long enough to know I had no choice in the matter, so I picked up the needle and wiggled around in the chair so I could line up my hand somewhat parallel to the pipe of a vein in front of me. I started to close my eyes but then quickly opened them. I had to keep my eye on the needle as it went into the vein, or it might go through the other side and cause a big hematoma. A freaky quote from Dave popped into my brain and distracted me momentarily. To him, baseball is full of metaphors for life: *Keep your eye on the ball, stupid!* And, lo and behold, it worked. I looked up just in time to see Dr. Sanders open his eyes, and we all broke out laughing. Eric pulled off the tourniquet, and we high-fived all around.

Now, one successful venipuncture does not guarantee you can do it again, so when I got to San Diego for the weekend, Dave, with a box in his hand, confronted me.

"Look what I brought home for you," he said, with love in his eyes.

To my dismay, Vampire Dave poured out at least a dozen butterfly needles, packaged alcohol swabs, and a beige tourniquet. What an awful way to spend the weekend.

"I can't do this to you!"

"Yes, you can, and you will. We're going to make sure you're good at this before you go back to LA next week."

I wanted to sit down and cry. He was right, though. The last thing I should be doing was practicing on patients who were sick and trusted me to take care of, not harm, them. So I rolled up to the kitchen table and locked my wheelchair.

"Okay, big boy. Let's see what you've got," I said. Dave made a fist and laid his arm out straight in front of me.

"When you get this side, then I want you to do the other arm," he said.

By Sunday night, I was pretty good at starting IVs, thanks again to my husband, who loves me and will do anything for me.

"Dr. Olson, please go to Dr. Sanders's office." The overhead announcement echoed throughout the radiology department. This was a common occurrence that struck fear in the hearts of all residents. I trundled to the back hallway and walked in with trepidation.

"Yes? What did I do?" This was my standard response to the command.

"Put your heart-shaped tush in that chair over there."

I let go of my cane and sat down. Dr. Sanders waited at his desk, twiddling something in his hands.

"When was your last menstrual period?"

"Pardon me? Why?"

"We need to figure out your exact due date to make sure it's well before the dates for the boards in Louisville."

Whew. I exhaled. *No problem there.* My due date was in early March, several months before the usual June exam dates. *I'll be svelte by then. None of those old geezer radiology examiners will know that I'm a new mom . . . and they'll pass me with flying colors. I'll soon be one of the boys, a board-certified radiologist.*

CHAPTER 7:

Building a House and Family

It was Friday night, and Dave was picking me up at the train station in Del Mar. As he put me in the car, he said, "Olsie, I don't know how we're going to do it, but we need to build a house."

I gulped when Dave looked at me and stated what had become obvious to both of us. While I was in LA, he rented the house that his parents owned but had left empty when Jack was stationed in Germany. Since all the bedrooms were upstairs, I had to pull myself, or he had to carry me, up and down, and I was definitely getting tired of it. Even though my paternal grandmother had told me my legs would grow back if we had faith and prayed hard enough, we knew the legless decades ahead of me would be much easier in a wheelchair-accessible home.

Weekends became a pain in the butt. We searched and searched for months, but there was no such thing as a ready-made wheelchair-accessible house. It was as if builders had put their heads in the sand and presumed everyone would always have two functioning legs. One step down into the living room. One step up into the kitchen. Three steps up to another level. Narrow halls. Even narrower doorways. Cramped bathrooms. What were all the old people doing? Did they just crawl into bed and never get out again? Where were all the wheelchair users? Were they locked up in facilities?

After six months, we finally found a piece of land we thought suitable for building. After working hard, studying every night, and trying to stay healthy for our unborn baby, I'd get off the train, go to Dave's parents' house, eat a quick supper, then sit at the dining room table with Dave and our architect, Jim.

It would start out amicably and then work its way to a fracas of some sort by the end of every meeting. We wanted something simple and affordable. The architect wanted an accessible showplace that would make the cover of an architectural publication, maybe *San Diego Home/Garden Lifestyles* magazine. We'd have preferred to move into a ready-made home; instead, we were obsessing over minutiae.

"Let's start with the living room tonight," Jim said as he pulled out new sketches.

"I don't think we need a living room. No one ever goes into living rooms anymore. Let's just have one big family-room space," I said nicely.

"I think you'll really like these windows," he said, ignoring my comment.

I leaned over the table to get a look at the plans. What I saw made no sense. Little, slit-like windows about twelve inches below the ceiling would provide the only light in the room.

"What are those things?" I asked. "They look like arrow slits in a fortress. They're really ugly." I minced no words. How could he be so stupid?

"Well, they'll give you privacy, and they're different, kind of cutting-edge-looking," he said, as if he were an architecture god.

"That's not happening," I said. I gritted my teeth and made a fist with my left hand under the table. Dave and I traded off trying to be civil as each encounter wore on.

As an amputee, I operated in two modes: one with my legs on, when I could walk using a cane in the house; the other when I left my prostheses off and rolled myself around in a manual wheelchair. This was very different from work, where I always walked with a cane. None of this appeared to be intuitive for Jim, so we put in hundreds of hours over the next several months, planning and making lists:

- things I did in my wheelchair;
- light switch placement;
- turning radius in every room;
- hallways and doorways wide enough for a wheelchair;
- pocket doors where possible;
- windows I could reach from wheelchair height and could open/close and lock/unlock with one hand;
- placement and distances for parts of the kitchen;
- lowering parts of the kitchen for me to work at;
- optimal height of the kick space under cabinetry, so I wouldn't catch my feet when I had my legs on;
- tile flooring choices, so I couldn't slip when walking;
- commercial-grade carpets, so my wheelchair would roll more easily;
- built-in bench seating on two sides of the kitchen table, which had to be bolted to the floor;
- flat doorway thresholds with adequate outdoor drainage so water wouldn't enter the house;
- and that eternal toilet problem—the right height, and something I could push off from so I could stand up.

After a full day strapped into my legs, I'd come home and ditch them as soon as possible. My wheelchair was best when I was at home. That at least made our building choices easier in some ways, but we were forced to put in an elevator because the lot we bought was so narrow that we had to build a two-story house.

While we prepared to build, I was incubating the baby that would make us a family. I couldn't wait for the house to become our home.

As I entered my last month of pregnancy, it became hard to concentrate and even harder to maneuver. I tried to be non-chalant when I talked to Dave during our nightly phone calls, but I knew he was worried about me, so I kept the calls short, hoping to sound cheery and upbeat.

"How's it going?" he asked one evening.

"Fine," I said. But, after a long pause, my stoicism crumbled, and I started to cry. "I can't do this anymore." My voice cracked, and I gripped the phone so tightly that my palm burned. "My legs itch all over, and my prostheses are so tight it's killing me to have them on all day."

"Olsie," Dave said in a firm voice, "it's time for you to come home. Your due date is a week away. I'm coming up tonight. I'll be there in a couple of hours. Pack your stuff, and we'll drive back down to San Diego in the morning."

I wanted to argue with him, to be tough, but I couldn't do it anymore. I needed to go home—or, rather, go to where Dave was living, the place where I could get lots of hugs while we waited together for the big event.

"Dave, wake up. What is *this*?" I whispered.

It was five o'clock in the morning on Thursday, March 12, 1981. My belly was big; my boobs were big; the baby rocking and rolling around in me felt big, too.

Dave turned on the bedside lamp and turned toward me. I ran my hand across the warm, wet bedsheets. No odor and no color. Amniotic fluid. Not much, just enough to know that today would be the day. We lay there a while longer, holding hands and squeezing our eyes shut, excitement and trepidation mounting.

"Come on. We might as well get up and see what happens," I mumbled.

Dave shoved me just enough that I didn't roll off onto the floor: turning over without legs while pregnant is like rolling a beach ball. We acted as though we were in a slow-motion movie, pretending to be calm, cool, and collected but all the while knowing that our lives were about to be changed unalterably again.

He called work and arranged to have someone else see his patients for the day while I showered and struggled to gussy up.

Just before we left, Dave got down on the floor to help me put on my legs, with the always-on brown knee-high leather boots that complemented the dark blue maternity dress stretched tightly over my abdomen.

It was late in the morning when we arrived at the labor-and-delivery deck of the Navy hospital. Only in the Navy would a pregnant woman go to a deck.

"Hey! Stop that lady with the boots! No boots on the labor deck!" the charge nurse yelled.

I looked around. *She's talking to me? You've gotta be kidding.* I didn't want to lose my balance by turning to look for her, but in my imagination I saw a stocky, militant woman with gray hair knotted tightly in a bun, surveying the mayhem with her clipboard as she roamed the hallways.

"Sorry. She's going in, boots and all. She can't walk without them."

Down the hall came a grinning Hugh Lacey, the ob-gyn chief resident who was scheduled to deliver our baby. His mild Southern drawl was disarming and always made me smile.

"Come on. Let's see how we're going to get this baby out!" he said as he greeted us in green scrubs and cap. His mask hung in front. Uncharted territory lay ahead.

A cheery young nurse created my room by yanking a yellow nylon curtain around the bed. Dave helped me pull off my dress and put on a hospital gown. Once dressed, I stood there looking at the nurse while I fiddled with the thin cotton covering that kept sliding off my armless right shoulder. The nurse waited for me to get up on the gurney bed, but it wasn't as if I could just rise up onto my tiptoes and slide backward, like most people. I'm not helpless, but I do need help with some things.

As if I were a feather, Dave set me up on the bed and kissed me at the same time, a skill he'd honed over the past year and a half. Now the experiments started. Because we were living one hundred miles apart, we did not attend any birthing classes. And there was no chapter in the obstetrical books about how to deliver a baby whose mom has no knees and no feet. I could hold my breath and grunt and exhale and create a great force, but without legs I had no way to translate all that hoopla into an effective push. It wasn't going to work if the stirrups at the end of the bed were empty. *I guess these fake legs are somehow going to have to come to life and do the job.*

For the first hour or two, it was relatively straightforward: blood pressure monitoring, manual cervical exam, normal stuff. As usual, I had a book with me, but it was hard to find time to read. Dave and Hugh hovered over me, stroking their chins, trying to imagine the perfect scenario for getting the baby out of me.

Then I started to squirm. I didn't want to sound wussy, so I just held my breath every time I felt a twinge. That didn't work for long.

"Dave, I'm getting a little uncomfortable."

"Breathe in and out through your mouth," he said, calm as could be. *Where does he get off telling me what to do? What I really want to do is YELL. AT. HIM. for getting me into this mess!*

"Ohhh-kaay," I said as I grimaced and grabbed the edge of the bed, looking down at the little mountain topped by the protuberant belly button that had replaced my flat abdomen. Below that, my boot-clad fake legs stretched out flat, the rigid, curved tops of my prostheses extending all the way up into my groin. Thigh-high nylons with lacy, patterned elastic tops added to the incongruity. I alternated between embarrassment and giggles, imagining how this appeared to other people.

Although mine was not technically a high-risk pregnancy, Hugh decided to give me an epidural, so I'd have energy to push later, and moved me into the delivery room "just in case." As they pushed me down the hall, my mind raced ahead of the gurney. *Will this be a pink or a blue? What if it's abnormal? I can barely take care of myself. . . . What if it dies? What if I die and Dave is left with it? I should never have agreed to keep it. I should have had an abortion. I shouldn't have added to Dave's lifetime burden.*

The physical demands of the present soon forced aside thoughts of the past and future.

"Push, push, push!" Hugh said. One man per leg, they leaned into my thighs, my left leg draped over Dave's shoulder, my right over Hugh's.

"Here, take this," Hugh commanded the attending nurse as he handed her my right leg. "I can feel the baby's head coming through your cervix, Linda. One more push for me. . . . Push!"

Within seconds, I heard a squeak of a cry as our new baby's lungs took over from the work of the placenta. I was an exhausted blob of happiness.

"You made a beautiful baby girl." Dave grinned at me through a veil of tears.

I smiled weakly.

"Cut the cord, Daddy," Hugh directed.

"Thank you, Hugh," I whispered. I was exhausted but managed a grin.

Baby Girl Hodgens was whisked off to the nursery, and Dave and I were spun down the hall to Recovery. Dave went out to accept hugs, cheers, and kisses from his family and Adrian and Johnny and to make the joyful call to my family. *Tomorrow, the three of us will start another life.* With that thought, I fell into a deep, exhausted sleep.

A couple of hours later, I was startled from my postpartum slumber by a nurse standing next to my bed. I blinked and tried to focus on what she was holding out to me. It was wrapped tightly in a blanket and wasn't very big. I strained to sit up but flopped back down.

The nurse looked at me, as if wondering why I wasn't reaching for the bundle. I gasped when I saw the gap between the bundle and my body.

"Wait! Can you pull the railings up on this bed? How am I going to hold that? It's going to roll off."

I felt as if she must be thinking, *My hands are full. Why don't you do that, lady?*

Frustrated, I grasped the right side of my gown to show her the emptiness where my arm should be. Her jaw dropped, and she stopped midtransfer.

"Oh! I'm so sorry . . . I didn't know. I'll be right back."

Before I knew what was happening, three angels in white uniforms appeared by my bed, straightened the sheets, surrounded me with pillows, raised the side rails, then tenderly propped a little baby girl on my right side while helping me turn so I could snuggle up to her. I wrapped my arm around her and buried my face in her neck.

"Thank you," I mumbled as they beamed at me and backed out of the room. I didn't move. I didn't know what to do. I was in limbo land. My pregnancy had been easy. I'd loved having that kicking, rolling baby inside me. In fact, I'd often thought it would be cool to have that sensation for the rest of my life. It was soothing, entertaining, and comforting all at once. I already missed it.

The baby squirmed and made a tiny sound. I felt frozen in place. *What is this thing? It's breathing, it's warm to the touch, it smells good. Why don't I know it? What's wrong with me?*

I leaned back and stared at the ceiling. My heart raced, and I felt faint. *Why did we do this?*

I looked down at her and whispered the name we'd chosen: "Tiffany."

Maybe it was my imagination, maybe not. She looked as if she'd heard me.

A little more loudly, I said, "Hi, puppy, it's your mom. How are you?"

Her eyes fluttered, and she puckered her rosebud lips. I reached over and gently pulled her onto my chest. Both of us closed our eyes and slept. We'd get to know each other in the morning.

~

"Come on, hon. I've got to get you out of here," Dave said.

With the charge nurse's permission, he parked illegally outside the maternity ward, ran up the stairs, swooped me into his arms, and carried me down the back stairs to the car. He then ran back up the stairs and returned with a nurse, who was carrying Tiffany and handed her to me.

Dave leaned over and kissed both his passengers before he started the engine. There were two new legs and two new arms in the car. We'd done it. We were going to have a normal life as a family, just like everyone else.

Five days later, Dave packed the car and took the first of thousands of trips to the beach at Scripps Pier. He parked at the top of the steep cement ramp that led to "our" beach. While I sat in the car, holding Tiffany, he hauled a diaper bag, two beach towels, and two chairs down to the sand and then returned to the car for us.

"Dave, how are you going to do this? We can't leave this tiny baby in the car while you carry me down."

"Hon," he said with a big grin, "lay Tiffany on the seat and put your arm around my neck."

Obediently, I put her down and reached up to encircle his neck with my left arm as he slid his right arm under my butt. In one deft move, he cradled Tiffany in his left arm, straightened up, and kicked the door shut with his foot.

"Wow, what a stud!" I said as he transported his family to their little beach sanctuary, where Tiffany would drink formula from a sandy bottle.

Two weeks after Tiffany was born, I returned to Los Angeles by myself to finish the last three months of my residency and take the American Board of Radiology oral exam.

Oral boards. The hardest, scariest, sweatiest, most gut-wrenching, most unpredictable examination of them all. Twenty years of studying and a couple hundred thousand dollars on the line. Your whole future hanging on this half-day test given once a year in Louisville. You walk into a hotel room and sit in front of a light box. The radiologist examiner gives you films and waits for you to describe them and then provide the correct diagnosis. In 1981, you did this seven times, then walked out and flew back home, chewing your nails and having stomach aches for a week while awaiting the results in the mail. I shrieked with joy when the letter arrived informing me that I'd passed. Tears of joy ran down my cheeks as I threw my arm around Dave and kissed him again and again. Thanks to him and our colleagues and friends, my dream had come true.

As a newly minted, board-certified radiologist, I had to find a job—a job in a specialty that had very few women. Of the 1.9 million people in San Diego County in 1981, there was only one woman in private-practice radiology and three at the University of California, San Diego. The prospect of a triple-amputee woman getting a job was almost nil.

Dave still had a two-year obligation to the Navy, so San Diego was the only reasonable place for me to look for a job.

In the two years since the accident, people in the radiology community had found out about me and were sympathetic, but sympathy doesn't get a contract. It just gets sympathy. And then one day, Jack Forrest, one of the senior members of the radiology department at UCSD, offered to share his office and suggested that I sit in on readouts in the chest section. About the same time, Dr. John Byfield, a radiation oncologist at UCSD, scrounged around and found $5,000 in an American Cancer Society grant, which became my salary that first year. The diagnostic radiology department worked with me to turn that into a year of computed tomography training.

During that year, I was given the chance to become part of the chest section. I will never forget watching a resident diagnose a small pneumothorax that I hadn't seen. I closed my eyes tightly, hoping to burn the image into my brain so I'd never miss a pneumothorax again. Back to the books I went, determined to become a good pulmonary radiologist.

I guess it worked, because in 1982 I was offered a full-time appointment in the radiology department at UCSD, a wonderful job that lasted for thirty years.

The end of my residency was also the end of my independent living in LA. While I adored our new baby and wanted to be with Dave full-time, the move back into his parents' two-story house was an ordeal. The only places open enough for me to maneuver in my manual one-arm-drive wheelchair were the family room and kitchen. No one in their right mind was going to carry that heavy wheelchair up and down the stairs every day. The bedrooms and full baths were on the second floor, which meant that when I had my legs on, I had to lever myself up and down the steps. Once I took them off at night, Dave had to carry me to the bathroom or from place to place, or I had to butt-walk around in the bedrooms. For me to change Tiffany's diaper or feed her or play with her, someone had to get her out of the crib and hand her to me while I sat on the floor or on the bed.

It became obvious that my new ticket to independence was now a wheelchair.

"Look what I can do," I said.

"Oh, no!" Dave's mom gasped the first time someone handed Tiffany to me while I sat in my wheelchair. I turned sideways a little, gently crammed her into the armless space along the right side, and leaned over to give her a big smooch on her forehead. With her little body snugged in by my hip and armrest, her head and neck supported by the backrest, she was like a papoose. She wasn't going anywhere. In fact, in all the years my two children were babies and toddlers, neither one ever fell out of my wheelchair. That's not to say that on occasion I didn't think about throwing them out.

For years, I mourned that I was unable to walk and hold my children's hands, not realizing the gift I'd been given, of having them sitting at my side in my wheelchair. While I cooked, did chores, did almost everything, they were snuggled up against me, until they were three or four years old. Another of life's silver linings.

The six months we lived with Dave's parents were a special time for all of us. In many ways, Tiffany's birth was a major landmark—we'd survived, and now we could thrive. We had accomplished many of our goals. I'd learned how to walk, returned to Los Angeles to live independently and finish my residency, and passed my boards. Now we were building a house where we'd be in charge of our lives again. But, perhaps most important, the gift of a new life helped Dave's parents as they took on their invaluable role as grandparents. We needed them, and they needed us.

Creating a family was one thing. Building the house was another. Excitement was high as we started: grading a lot that had never been built on, placing the forms, and pouring the concrete foundation, with parts of pipes that would eventually become plumbing and electricity sticking up. My favorite part was the framing—smelling the wood and seeing the ghosts of rooms appear as the two-by-four Douglas fir studs went up. Why can't houses smell like that for the next twenty-five years? I loved looking out of the rectangular spaces that would become windows and doors and skylights, places that would bring the outdoors in.

Summer turned into fall. Things slowed down. If we dropped by unexpectedly, we might or might not find workers on-site. The promise of a house in six months dragged into nine, essentially another pregnancy. By Thanksgiving, the workers stopped coming to work, and by mid-December, our dream of a family Christmas in our home was fading fast. The only leverage we had was withholding the final payments the contractor was requesting.

"We need to move in," Dave said one night.

"Are you crazy?" I said. "There's no electricity and no hot water."

"Well, we can just pretend we're camping," he said.

"Hmm, I've camped a lot in my life . . . Why not?"

Dave continued, "I'll take our mattress and a camp stove down there after work tomorrow. I've talked to my folks, and they said they're happy to keep Tiffany here with them. You and I are going to start living down there."

Now you're talking. I felt myself start to smile.

For the first few nights, we didn't have electricity, but one toilet had been installed, so we were able to get by without using the port-a-potty or digging a hole in the backyard. It was almost civilized. We would come home from work, eat dinner at Dave's parents' house, play with Tiffany, put her to bed, then drive five miles to our dark house. We would park in front, and Dave would haul me up the steps. While I held a flashlight, he'd carry me into our bedroom and set me down on the bed. We were so tired that we were asleep within minutes.

Early each morning, we drove back up to Dave's parents' house, took showers, got ready, and went to work. This got our contractor's attention. That and the fact that we were withholding his last payment, the payment he needed to pay his employees and suppliers.

"Let's have Christmas dinner here," I said one morning. "After all, this is our house and we're in charge here."

Dave looked at me for a minute, then said, "Why not? We can make the food at my folks' house, bring it down, and warm it on hot plates."

And so a large piece of plywood set on sawhorses became our first dining room table. Folding chairs, paper plates, silver utensils, red candles, and a pine-bough centerpiece in an otherwise empty house became our first Denver Street Christmas dining display. My parents and brother and sister joined Dave's family in celebrating family, love, and renewal of the human spirit.

We completed our move the first week in January. Our new, king-size mattress was already directly on the floor, without a frame. This allowed me to get down out of my wheelchair easily so I could butt-walk around and play with Tiffany as she learned to crawl and walk. My old college dorm collection of orange crates, concrete cinder blocks, and painted one-by-six boards became our bedroom bookshelves. A set of drawers was already built in next to the closet. Two large papasan chairs sat in the otherwise empty family room. Tiffany's crib and a small changing table went into her room. It wasn't fancy, but it was home.

Our hodgepodge kitchenware was quickly hidden away in the cupboards. Our nice china dishes and crystal remained packed away in boxes and stored at Dave's parents' house. The kitchen table was built in with bench seating on two sides, leaving the other sides open for my wheelchair so I could sit down easily with or without my legs. It also took up less space and kept me from having to deal with chairs getting in my way.

The custom-built dining area was almost perfect.

"I've got it," Dave exclaimed one evening. A big grin lit up his face.

"Got what?" I said.

"The perfect piece of furniture that will make your life amazing!"

This sounded unbelievable, but was I ever wrong. Dave's second furniture brainchild became the centerpiece of my life for several years. The eight-by-four-foot table he designed and built was covered with foam and Naugahyde and occupied a corner of our otherwise empty dining room. With two sides butted up against walls, this utilitarian, wheelchair-height platform became Tiffany's changing table, my exercise mat, and the space where I could wrassle with Tiffany and later Brian. It was also the place for my peculiar one-handed, pat-it-out-and-pretend-it's-ironed form of finishing the laundry.

In keeping with our wish to be outdoors as much as possible, the first real furniture we bought was a patio table and chairs. Over the next five years, we built a garage and furnished one room at a time, only as we could pay for them.

Now that the house had become our home, we set about creating our oasis. No doorbell and an unlisted phone number were idiosyncrasies we became known for. After busy days at work, we craved peace and quiet. We indulged in our love of music, morning-time Bach and Mozart, and jazz after work in the evenings: Brubeck, Shearing, Bolling, Davis, Hancock—names from our parents' generation that we passed on to our children. TV was outlawed in the family room. Instead, a big sheepskin rug in front of the fireplace became our refuge for reading to the kids and getting them ready for bed. Many times Dave carried them asleep up the stairs and put them gently into bed without their awakening. They loved it as much as he did.

Having graduated from college and medical school in the '70s, I was on the front edge of the "supermom" era—a term Merriam-Webster's dictionary says was first used in 1974, when I was halfway through medical school. The dictionary defines it as "a woman who performs the traditional duties of housekeeping and child-rearing while also having a full-time job." I realized pretty early on that being a supermom was next to impossible for me. My disability was severe enough that I would need housekeeping and childcare help, even if I didn't work.

When I got home from work, I often lingered in my car in the garage—the in-between zone for me. My "doctor" workday done, I readied for my "mom" time. Dinner, homework, chores, the family together. There was a sameness to my "doctor" day. "Mom" time evolved as our children got older and their needs changed, from diaper changing and lullabies to wrassling and homework, then on to sports activities and dating. I suspect that all families with two working parents worry about the time they do or don't spend with their children. "Quality time" was a popular catchphrase. Was this a rationalization for spending less time with our children than we spent at work? Were my kids glad I wasn't home with them, or did they feel neglected?

I realized pretty early on that being a supermom was next to impossible. There was no way I could ever have been one. Just being a good mom was hard enough, but it *is* enough.

To my dismay, I found myself waking at night, haunted by more issues. Motherhood was wonderful but made me very dependent again. I was physically unable to care for my baby by myself. This put more responsibility on Dave. I'd come to realize that my role at work was just the opposite. I was most independent and functional when I was there. I needed very little assistance and was just as efficient as my colleagues. It seemed to me that I should take advantage of working, because it was where I was most productive, yet I knew the importance of motherhood and being a wife would outweigh my job in the long run. I wanted to be engaged with both: work and normal mom stuff.

Childcare. Driving a car. Keeping house. For my sanity, we needed to prioritize our needs.

Not long after I started mentally prioritizing things, Dave, ever the list maker, said, "Olsie, have you thought of the lists we made when we were in Salzburg?"

"No, not recently."

"Well, I have. In fact, I found them in a three-ring binder the other day. Wanna see 'em?"

I knew exactly what he was referring to. Everything he'd done that first year, he had duly typed up and placed chronologically in a utilitarian blue cloth binder. He'd done much of it while I was still in the hospital. Seven of the pages were from the first week in Salzburg. Two pages were Dave's—in his normal, tiny, hard-to-read, classic doctor penmanship. The five in my new, awkward left-hand print were partly handwriting practice and partly a detailed wish list for my unasked-for new life.

I pushed myself over to his desk and saw his list first:
Problems to solve:

Place to live in San Diego
Transportation
Bathing, toilet
Communication
Kitchen

My list was longer and went into more detail. In fact, four of my pages spelled out the issues and what I thought might be solutions. The first page was the shortest:

Personal
Rehabilition [sic]
Proffessional [sic]
Socially
Marital
Family
Psycological [sic] adjustment
Sports activities
~~Occupational adjustments~~
Desirable goals: drive

We were quiet as we looked at each page. In the two years and five months since the accident, we'd worked hard and accomplished many of our goals. Noticing the misspellings on my pages reminded me of how disorienting it had been to start writing with my nondominant left hand. I paused to remember how scared I'd been seeing all the incorrect words, how I'd had to force myself to spell words out loud to correct them, how I'd wondered if I'd ever be able to spell easily again.

Dave took my hand and placed it between his two strong ones. "I'm so proud of you. You've—"

"Wait," I said. "Stop saying *you*. It's *us*. We've done this together."

I realized that while we had crossed off many of the things on our lists, we weren't finished. I still couldn't drive. And if I couldn't drive, I couldn't be a "normal" mom.

The Night Shift

I hear the sound I wait for, even in my sleep. The baby is crying. Tiffany. She's only a few weeks old and still so small that her cries, although persistent, are soft. They are demanding but not unpleasant, and I know they are as strong as her little lungs and larynx can make them. Cries of need. Cries of vulnerability.

Instinctively I rise, slip on the jeans that are beside the bed, and make my way through the 2:00 a.m. darkness, taking care not to wake Linda. I sneak barefoot into the otherwise quiet bedroom that holds the crib and gently grasp the crying infant, with one hand behind her head and the other holding her firm little body, and revel in the feeling of cuddling her up to my chest. She's still crying, with her eyes closed, but this is the best. I know she probably needs a diaper change and feeding. I will take care of those things momentarily, but this holding is the reward. My baby. Our baby. There is no joy in the world that is so heavy. Linda, dear Linda, has kept her promise to me, and I know I must continue to keep my promise to her, and now to Tiffany.

Linda knew my feelings about kids long before we got married. I love them. I grew to love them during every pediatric rotation I did in medical school. The pediatric nurses in the hospital, from the neonatal ICU up to the wards, loved me because I would hold the sick children, care about them, and empathize with their agonized parents. I found them so easy to care for and care about. Holding a sick child and helping soothe it through its illness was one of the most fulfilling experiences I ever had. The worst were on the pediatric psych rotation, where I saw what happened when kids had only part of a parent, or none at all.

I quickly got used to the secretions and the excretions and the vomitus that might come forth, so I wasn't squeamish in the least. These were innocent, sick children suffering from illnesses they could never understand, and thus represented the ultimate in vulnerability. I could easily have spent a happy career as a pediatrician. So I wanted to be a dad. Especially to Linda's children.

"I know what you want," Linda said when I realized she was pregnant. But then concern took over. "Can we do this? Is this a good time? Will I be able to keep walking? Will I be able to work?" The glowing skin of her face betrayed well-founded anxiety. She fixed her gaze on my eyes and held me to account.

I knew what that look meant. It was the unspoken question. It was the same unspoken question she had transmitted to me from the bed in the

ICU after the accident. Put into words, which are far less powerful than the look, the question was: Will you be there? Will you stay with me? Will you help me? Will you run away? *And now:* Will you help me with pregnancy and a baby and a child and a lifetime of parenthood?

"*I will be here for you, and for our baby, and for other babies, and for our children as they grow. I will do anything and everything that's necessary to make this work. I will get up at night and feed and change diapers. You know how I feel about kids and about wanting a family, and about you,*" *I said as I reached to wipe a tear that had rolled down her cheek.*

"*Okay,*" *she whispered, and smiled.*

The bond between us forged another link. We would do this.

Clean, dry, powdered, and wearing a new diaper, Tiffany is suckling down the last half ounce of her half bottle. I've got her wrapped up in a comfy, soft cotton blanket, and she is resting in my arms as I sit in the easy chair. She is beginning to suck a little less vigorously, and her eyes are closed, and I know that she will be asleep in a few minutes. I give her a gentle squeeze and a light kiss on the forehead as she finishes her bottle. I hold her upright, with her face near a towel on my shoulder, and pat her gently on the back until she has released the air she has swallowed and is completely at ease. But I will enjoy the holding of my baby for a while longer before I put her back down and make her comfortable in the crib and then sneak back into our bedroom. I know that I will be tired tomorrow, and maybe for the rest

*of my life. I know also that I am a lucky man. I'm
Dad. As with the other promises I made to Linda,
this will be an easy one to keep.*

*I listen for the sound that I know to wait for, even
in my sleep. It's Brian crying. I slip out of bed and
into my jeans and sneak out of the bedroom and
quietly close the door. I find the source of the soft
cries and happily pick him up and hold him to my
chest. He'll need the usual change and feeding, but
this is the best. I love this feeling. It is as soothing
to me as it is to him. I can keep him warm, make
him comfortable, and satisfy his need for food. It
is quiet. It is the middle of the night. There are no
distractions. My wife and daughter are asleep and
safe and undisturbed. I can enjoy these moments of
holding my baby. Our baby. I say a silent prayer of
thanks to Linda the Indomitable. The future, for
now and for us, is just the next feeding. And right
now, I'm just Dad. No other joy is this heavy.*

Chapter 8:

Look, Ma, No Feet

······································

As Dave opened the passenger-side door and slid into our car, I sidled up to the driver's seat, turned, and plopped down. My rigid fake legs and feet hung outside the car. Grasping the bottom of my pant leg, I pulled my right leg up and swung it into the car and then, like a marionette puppeteer, did the same with the left leg. It was good to sit in the driver's seat again and put my hand on the steering wheel.

In my head, I could hear the voice of my driver's ed instructor yelling at the sixteen-year-old me for the umpteenth time: *Ten and two . . . Come on, let's get those hands at ten and two.* I wondered what he'd say to one-armed me.

"Okay," I said, with a smirk on my face. "If that's all it takes, I can do it."

My attempt at humor masked the churning in my stomach. What if we couldn't figure out a way for me to drive? Being unable to do so would be a knockout punch that would compound my disability.

Dave sat in the front passenger seat, trying to exude optimism. Tiffany was a year old, and I'd finished my residency and was doing a fellowship in radiology at UCSD, with an offer for a one-year position there. In the two and a half years since the accident, I'd never driven anywhere by myself. I always sat in the passenger seat.

There was a lot riding on this. To hold down a job, I had to be able to get to work reliably, which would occasionally be in the middle of the night if I was called to go in to the hospital. I also needed to be a mommy chauffeur, trucking Tiffany and any kids who followed to school, doctor's appointments, sports, and social activities. I wanted to do the grocery shopping by myself, maybe on the way home from work, maybe late in the evening, after the kids had gone to bed. And, last but not least, I wanted to pull my weight so Dave wouldn't be handicapped in his career or his personal life by being the only driver in the family.

"Okay, this seems doable. I think you'll need a . . . What's the name of it? You know, the suicide-knob thing?" Dave asked.

"A necker knob, or a granny knob," I said. *Sheesh*. Stump, suicide, *and* granny knobs. *Who makes up words?* "It's not the steering that concerns me. It's these legs that I don't know about."

"Move the seat up and see if you can get your foot on the gas pedal," Dave said.

I lifted my right leg and was rewarded by nothing more than the rigid plastic thigh moving up. My foot was nowhere near the gas pedal. Wiggling my thigh up and down and side to side did not get the fake foot any closer to the pedal. So, again, I leaned over, grabbed my lower pant leg, pulled the foot up, and flopped it onto the gas pedal. So far, so good. But that was the end of it.

When I tried to move it to the brake pedal, it just hung suspended in air. Letting go of the steering wheel to grab my pant leg and reposition my foot wasn't going to cut it. I wanted to pull off the worthless fake legs and throw them as far as I could, watch them fly off into the wild blue yonder, where they'd be as useless as they were here.

"Why couldn't I have lost just one leg? Think of all the things I could still do with one leg and one arm."

I tried to push down the frustration and fear that were rising to the surface in the form of hot tears.

Dave leaned across the center console, kissed my neck, and said, "We'll figure it out. At least you have the prescription so we can get what we need to adapt the car. Let's see what they say."

⁓

A few days later, prescription in hand, we entered the Sharp Rehab Center for an appointment with Sandy Bartlow, a driving rehab specialist. I walked in with my quad cane and distinctive toy-soldier gait, hoping she'd see how strong and accomplished I was.

"I must admit that you are a challenge. Most of our patients are paraplegics or stroke victims, and while they have weak or paralyzed limbs, at least they have four extremities for us to work with. I've never seen a triple amputee, let alone had one try to drive."

My firm handshake got her attention. "Well, that arm is certainly strong," she said.

She had many concerns. Was my core strength adequate for sitting, steering, and using a gas-brake device? Could I turn my head to see behind me? Was my arm strong enough to steer? Had I ever driven before? Did I have head trauma? Could I pass the driving test?

"A person needs two extremities to drive, one for steering and the other for gas and brake. Right?" I asked.

"Yes," she answered. "The typical adaptive driving setup is a lever on the steering column for gas and brake, with a spinner knob on the steering wheel for turning. Then the controls for headlights, turn signals, windshield wipers, and horn need to be located so you can reach them with whichever residual hand you have. Let's go sit in the driver's-ed car and see what you can do."

I gamely opened the car door, sat down, and rolled my eyes at Dave. In less than two minutes, Sandy knew there wasn't an off-the-shelf device for me.

"Is there a company in town that does adaptive work on vehicles? Would it help to go talk to them and see if they have any ideas?" I asked.

"The big question is, are you going to need a wheelchair all or most of the time? If so, we should put you in a van so you can drive while sitting in it."

It sounded as though Sandy thought this might be my only solution.

"I want to drive a car, just like everyone else," I said.

"In that case," she said, "I think we should go to a company over on Ronson Road."

I closed my eyes and fought the dark, bottomless pit inside me as Dave drove me home.

George Hendrickson was a paraplegic World War II vet who, with Butch Lee, started manufacturing hand-control devices for paraplegics. We hit it off immediately. George seemed to be in charge. He was a salty character with a twinkle in his eyes and a joke for everything. His graying blond hair, weathered face, and gravelly voice belied his heart of gold. He made me feel attractive and maybe even a little sexy. Butch was more reserved and slightly dour. His flat-top haircut was vintage '50s. Their work uniform seemed to be white T-shirts and faded blue jeans. Together, their brains and brawn had given the gift of mobility to hundreds of disabled people years before the Americans with Disabilities Act.

After the initial pleasantries and jocularity, I sat down in the driver's seat of our car and watched George as he rolled up in his sleek, low-slung wheelchair. He parked as close to me as he could get.

"Okay," he said. "Let's see what you can do. I want you to get comfortable." He reached down for the seat lever. "Move the seat to a position where you can rest your hand easily on the steering wheel."

I tried to move the seat forward. Nothing happened. I tried to jump a little to move the seat forward. Still nothing.

George straightened up. "You're going to need a power seat, power windows and door locks and power steering, and an automatic transmission. It's pretty expensive to get all this stuff."

I felt as if we'd slammed into the first roadblock at sixty miles per hour.

Dave reacted first. "Looks like we need to buy a new car before we go any further." He turned to George. "What would you suggest? What makes or models work best for the equipment you need to put in them?" After some discussion, George told us to look at Oldsmobiles and see if we could drive one back to Manufacturing & Production Services (MPS) for their approval before we completed the purchase.

"Well, let's do what we can today. Will you be wearing your artificial legs when you drive?"

I hadn't thought about that.

"Hmm, it would be nice to be able to drive with or without them," I said. After thinking for a second, I added, "Actually, I'll need to have them on if I'm not using a wheelchair, and I don't want to have to use a wheelchair, so with, I guess."

"Okay. Get yourself settled in whatever position you're most comfortable in; then I want you to plant your heels on the floor and swivel your knee sideways, back and forth—only one to two inches each way."

He watched my every move with the eyes and mind of an engineer.

"Hey, Butch. Come over and take a look. I'm thinking we could bastardize one of our hand-control devices, somehow mount it under the seat and connect it to her right knee. Maybe she could activate the gas while pushing out and the brake by pulling in with her knee. What do you think?"

Later that week, Dave drove me back to MPS in a brand-new Oldsmobile Omega. Our foursome gathered in the parking lot to do a final assessment. George rolled out of the way so Butch could lean in and assess the situation. He felt the space under the driver's seat. I blushed, even though my fake legs couldn't feel his touch, when he put his head between them to look under the dashboard to make sure he had room to install the mechanical parts.

"Yeah, I think we can do something. Maybe fabricate a metal yoke that will cradle her knee so she gets gas and brake with small, back-and-forth, sideways movements," Butch said to George.

As he straightened up, he eyeballed the interior of the car. His mechanic's mind was looking at the location of all the functions I'd need to be able to reach with my left hand: headlight high beams and dimmer, horn, windshield wipers, and turn signals. He hesitated as he looked at the gearshift lever on the right side of the steering column.

"Can you reach the gearshift lever?" he asked. "You're going to have to let go of the steering wheel and stick your hand through it to move the lever up and down when you put it in reverse or park."

I had a small panic attack but then realized that with an automatic gear shift, I would change gears only when the car was at a standstill, so steering shouldn't be a problem.

"Well," Butch said as he turned toward George, "this just might work. It'll be a one-of-a-kind installation."

He winked as he stood up and said, "I just don't want to see you waving at people as you're turning corners." I wanted to smother them with hugs and kisses.

My driving lessons took place with Sandy and Dave in the parking lot of Jack Murphy Stadium, at that time the home of the Padres and Chargers, San Diego's professional baseball and football teams.

Holding the key with my left hand, I twisted my wrist around, trying to insert the key into the ignition on the right side of the steering column. It didn't work—I couldn't turn it far enough. Leaving the key in the ignition, I repositioned my hand. Several times.

"Damn it," I said. "This should be the simple part." I finally found the right angle, and with a firm push, I started the engine. What a marvelous sound! This was going to work.

My mind knew how to drive. Using one hand for what would normally have been two hands was fairly straightforward. It just required attention to detail and crossing my hand back and forth quickly. With fifteen years of driving under my belt, I knew it should be just a matter of mastering the brake and acceleration functions with my knee instead of my foot. It seemed to me that the fright reaction would be to pull in, so braking became the inward motion. That left gas as the outward knee push. Intellectually, this made perfect sense. Until I tried it.

The engine was running. I was comfortably seated. I looked around. The vast stadium parking lot was empty, a mile of asphalt around me. One more glance right to left.

"Okay, Linda, give it a try." Dave's voice was quiet and patient. Leaving the gearshift lever in park, I pulled in with my knee and watched the brake pedal depress. I pushed out and heard the engine rev into a roar. *Oops, that was a bit much.* Good thing I was still in park; otherwise, we'd have catapulted over the stadium. I did it again. This time, almost nothing.

"Dave, this is really weird. I can't feel anything. I can tell my leg is moving, but I have no idea how much."

A driving demon howled inside me, *Ha, you can't do it.* I tried again, this time so gently and slowly that my leg quivered. No acceleration. *What's wrong? There's no sensation. This is a problem.*

I sat still and tried to clinically think my way through the challenge. Putting my hand on my thigh, I pushed it from side to side. Why, of course! My proprioception was way off-kilter. In fact, my feet proprioceptors were totally gone.

Wikipedia defines proprioception as "the sense of the relative position of neighboring parts of the body and strength of effort being employed in movement." It goes on to state:

> The brain integrates information from propriocep-
> tion and from the vestibular system into its overall
> sense of body position, movement, and acceleration.
> Proprioception is what allows someone to learn to
> walk in complete darkness without losing balance.
> During the learning of any new skill, sport, or art,
> it is usually necessary to become familiar with some
> proprioceptive tasks specific to that activity. Without
> the appropriate integration of proprioceptive input,
> an artist would not be able to brush paint onto a
> canvas without looking at the hand as it moved the
> brush over the canvas; it would be impossible to
> drive an automobile because a motorist would not
> be able to steer or use the pedals while looking at

the road ahead; a person could not touch-type or perform ballet; and people would not even be able to walk without watching where they put their feet.

In addition to major proprioception deficits, I had essentially put my residual leg inside a tight-fitting tin can and then pushed the can against a metal lever. I couldn't sense how much brake or acceleration I'd get each time until after I'd pushed it and the car started moving. Plus, sensations from my skin were missing because I was encased in the "can." This would be a new experiment every time I started the car and got situated.

Oh well—I'd just have to get over it and make it work.

Ten years later, I returned to the stadium parking lot to practice using a different adaptive driving device, one that the Ability Center had installed in my new, blue Taurus station wagon. A lot had changed. Dave was in the front passenger seat, but our eleven-year-old daughter and eight-year-old son were passengers in the back seat. They were by then accustomed to their mom's automobile idiosyncrasies: air-conditioning always on full blast, Christmas music blaring in July, obsession with putting the turn signal on way before the turn.

Dave had taught them handicapped-placard etiquette and how to deal with obtuse drivers who park in handicapped spots "for just a minute to run in."

"We never park in blue spots unless Mom is getting out of the car. When you are parked there, a person who needs it can't park there."

"Come on, Mom," Tiffany said. "Hit the gas! Why are you going so slow?"

"Yeah," Brian echoed. "Show us what you can do."

I pushed out with my right thigh, and the car shot forward across the vast, empty lot, wind blowing our hair. When I looked in the rearview mirror, I saw that the kids had outfitted themselves in elbow and knee pads and batting helmets advertising 31 Flavors and the San Diego Padres. They looked as if they were having the time of their lives, flopping around as if they were going to fly out of the car at any second.

I pulled a little more strongly than necessary on the brake and snuck another look back at them. Their eyes got really big, and they shrieked even more loudly as they rolled around in the back seat. We laughed so hard that by the time the car stopped, tears were running down our cheeks.

Years later, I still feel an adrenaline rush as I cruise down Torrey Pines Road—the giddy sense of freedom and happiness I get every day as I drive alone, going wherever I want, whenever I want. I never take driving for granted. It is my equalizer. It lets me forget for a while the things I can't do, lets me be a productive, normal person.

With a new house, a new baby, prospects for a new job, and my first adaptive driving device, I knew normalcy was within reach.

CHAPTER 9:

Tits and Ass

....

"Tiffany," I called out. "Daddy's ready to go."

I heard our two-year-old run out of her room and come bouncing down the stairs to where I sat in my wheelchair. She loved going to Grandma and Grandpa Hodgens's house with its huge backyard and garden. In particular, she loved Grandpa's wheelbarrow. It was a cherished sight to see him pushing and careening around the yard while she shrieked and yelled, "Faster, Grandpa. Go faster!"

"I'm glad your parents are in such good shape," I said to Dave. "She'd wear them out if they weren't."

He kissed my forehead and, with a dramatic swoop, scooped Tiffany up into his arms and halfway over his shoulder. He blew her blond hair out of his face as she kicked and giggled and leaned toward the door.

After they left, I let out a big sigh of relief and turned to packing my suitcase: a dress for eating out at the nice restaurants we'd already chosen, jeans for most of our sightseeing in Santa Barbara and at the Santa Ynez Valley wineries we hoped to visit, a bathing suit in case there was a hot tub, and my skimpy lingerie.

As the road stretched out ahead of us and San Diego shrank in the rearview mirror, Dave unwound more and more. His goofy, let's-have-fun side eclipsed his no-nonsense, get-things-done side. It reminded me of the feelings I'd had years before on the beach near Punta Estrella, Mexico.

"I think this is it," Dave said as he parked and we got out of the car. The sun warmed my skin, and the sky reflected endless possibilities. A relatively flat dirt trail headed into a shady, wooded area. I gripped Dave's rigidly flexed right arm with my left arm and leaned on him as I hiked using my prostheses. When I got tired, I draped my arm over his shoulders and he carried me. We were young and strong enough to do the half-mile walk alternating between my walking and his carrying me.

Our effort was rewarded when we reached our destination and looked at the ancient pictographs of Chumash Painted Cave through the protective grate. Dave stood quietly, taking it all in. After several minutes, he turned and asked, "Can you imagine what it was like to be an Ice Age caveman living among saber-toothed cats and dire wolves?"

"Nope," I said as I put my arm around his neck and purred, "How about 'Me Tarzan, you Jane'?"

"Ooh . . . Now, that's nice," he whispered in my ear.

Rests on the way back were frequent because the walking and carrying were difficult.

"I've got to put you down for a minute," Dave said.

The woods were quiet, and all my day-to-day distractions had melted away. I noticed every fiber of Dave's hard muscles as he lowered me to the uneven ground and jogged off-trail.

"Be right back," he said over his shoulder before disappearing into the woods.

Running back to me with a big grin on his face, he picked me up and carried me into the trees. My braless boobs jiggled against him, and I kissed the back of his neck as he hauled me to a big, flat granite slab. From our spot, which was completely hidden from the trail, we had a beautiful view out to the north, over a canyon. The midday sun warmed us as I snuggled up against him.

"Mmm," he said. "You feelin' friendly?"

"Mm-hmm. Me hot little cavewoman," I murmured with a throaty giggle.

"I like being alone with you in the woods," he whispered.

I looked into his green eyes and held his gaze as he kissed me on the lips. Then we melted into each other in our ancient rock boudoir. Afterward, we lay quietly, basking in the afterglow. I could have stayed there forever.

The Chumash Painted Cave State Historic Park website has this to say: "We are working to improve accessibility throughout our parks, but we regret that there are currently no accessible activities at this park." Dave and I beg to differ!

Our son, Brian, was born nine months later.

Every year on Brian's birthday, Dave gets a sly grin on his face, and I know he's daydreaming about our romantic interlude on that big, flat rock.

~

Pregnancy was less intimidating the second time around, but no less entertaining. In the four years since the accident, both Dave and I had secured stable jobs that we liked, and externally our life was reasonably normal. We'd also found a way to hire a live-in nanny-housekeeper, who was a real sweetheart.

"Michelle, I'm ready," I'd call out every morning. Then I'd sit in my wheelchair and wait for her to come around the corner and into our bedroom with her usual smile.

"How are you feeling today?" she always asked.

"Darn good" was my standard answer, and the one I gave her one day during my third trimester.

She sighed and put her hand on the edge of the dresser as she knelt to help me put on my legs. "My, my," she said, with a little giggle, "I can finally tell you're pregnant. Your ankles are starting to swell."

"Uh, Michelle . . . these legs are fake. I don't think they can swell."

She looked confused for a second, then flushed, and then we burst out laughing.

As Brian's due date approached, it got hard to sleep. Every morning I whispered to myself, "Today would be a good day to have a baby."

Monday, March 26, started like all the rest. We got up, made breakfast, fed Tiffany, and went to work.

I parked in my reserved spot, grabbed hold of my legs, and swung them out of the car. I slung my briefcase over my shoulder, grabbed the railing, pulled myself up the three steps that led to the west entrance of the Hillcrest hospital, and plodded down the long, deserted hallway. My *thump-thud* toy-soldier walk was slow and laborious, and I stayed close to the right wall, just in case I started to lose my balance. I stopped several times to catch my breath before I finally reached my office and fell into my chair. I shuffled piles of paper around on my desk, trying to triage what needed doing and what I could ignore.

I lumbered over to the main reading room, sat at the ICU board, and prepared to read the morning films on the hospital's sickest patients, those in the intensive care units. Many of my colleagues considered this a mundane chore, but it was a morning ritual I'd come to appreciate *because* of its routineness. After a few days, the sickest patients became familiar, and as I watched their ups and downs, I hoped each morning to see them improve and move on out to the regular floors. I was saddened on the mornings when I saw a chest X-ray hanging upside down—a sign from the overnight house staff that the patient hadn't made it.

I switched on the alternator lights, looked at the first set of films, and, somewhat short of breath, started dictating. *I can do this. Don't quit yet. Remember what Barbara said: "Don't let people think you're lazy or a slacker." Now of all times, I've got to pull my weight, got to be a good example. I'm a woman, I'm disabled, and I'm pregnant . . .*

By 5:00 p.m., I was ready to call it a day. I trudged back to my office and plopped down with a big sigh. The piles of paperwork hadn't disappeared. In fact, there were more than when I'd started that morning. It was as if they'd been mating and reproducing right on my desk. They'd just have to wait.

"Good night, Lee," I said to Dr. Talner, my friend and colleague, as I locked my door and started down the hall to my car.

By 6:00 p.m., I was home and getting ready to make dinner when I felt the first convincing contraction. I took a deep breath and waited. Another. And then another.

"Dave, what are you doing?" I asked as I continued tearing up lettuce with my one hand.

"Nothing," he said.

"You should make yourself a drink."

"Why should I make myself a drink?"

"Well, I'm starting to have contractions."

"What? The last thing I need is a drink! How far apart are they?"

Within minutes, it was clear that we needed to get going.

"Go ask Michelle to feed Tiffany. I'm going to go pack my bag," I said.

As we waited for the elevator near the front desk of the radiology department, I waved at the evening desk clerk and, with a sheepish grin, told him we were going upstairs to have a baby. And that's exactly what happened. Brian was born at 9:15 p.m., not four hours after I'd left work. Just before midnight, Dave kissed me good night; hoisted my legs, with the pants still on, over his head; and draped them around his shoulders to make the walk down the same long, deserted hallway I'd traveled early that morning.

Guess I showed them. I'm not a slacker.

The year was 1984. There was no pregnancy leave policy in my department, so my pregnancy and postpartum leave were without precedent. Eager to return to the place I felt most useful, I took only one month away from the office, but not away from work. As a faculty member in the chest section for almost three years, I'd been given my first big lecture assignment, speaking at the Radiology Residents Review Course on mediastinal anatomy and diseases. This was to take place about six weeks after I gave birth to Brian. We thought it reasonable that I take four weeks' maternity leave, time I could use to practice my talk for the radiology resident review course. I took rehearsing for this talk seriously. I look back on that interlude as the basis for my career as a teacher, which eventually included many teaching awards.

My two physician role models for teaching and lecturing were my father, who was a pathologist at Loma Linda University School of Medicine, and my radiology residency program director, Ike Sanders. As a child in the '60s, I watched my father put the slides in a Kodak carousel, set up his projector in his and my mom's bedroom, and project the slides on the white, sliding closet door. He practiced his lectures until they were perfect. He left nothing to chance. My radiology mentor, Dr. Sanders, taught me to "tell them what you're going to tell them, tell them, then tell them what you told them." He also insisted that every talk be timed so it didn't go over the allotted interval.

UCSD was one of the first radiology departments to create a review course to help prepare radiology residents for the American Board of Radiology oral exam. In fact, I'd been one of about five hundred anxious senior residents attending the course the second year it was offered. Residents from all over the country squeezed shoulder to shoulder at long tables in a darkened hall from 7:00 a.m. until sometimes 8:00 p.m. for six days. Hundreds of X-ray images flashed on enormous screens in the front of the hall while we scribbled copious notes in the dark, hoping that we could regurgitate the pearls being presented by the time we arrived in Louisville a few weeks later. But it was more than just test taking that weighed on us. This was information that would translate into patient care for the rest of our professional lives. I had been in awe of the UCSD professors' well-prepared and pertinent lectures. It was a dream come true to be one of them now.

My lack of extremities seemed less important as I settled into my role as a radiologist, however, my missing limbs became more obvious as our family life evolved.

Giggles first, then shrieks of laughter emanated from our bedroom. It was wrassle time, my favorite time of the day. Coming home after a long day at work and pulling off my fake legs, I entered the oasis of our home. No matter how tired I was, seeing my children run toward me energized me for at least three more hours every evening.

Wheeling myself to the edge of our king-size bed, I butt-walked onto it as the kids ran around the corner and flung themselves onto the mattress. Rolling over, I grabbed them with my arm, pulled them up tightly onto my chest, and squeezed them with my short amputated legs. Then I rolled back and forth until we were laughing so hard we couldn't breathe. It annoyed the heck out of them until they were about three or four years old and could break free from my bear hug of a grip on them.

As they got older and could walk and run, the next game evolved: butt-walk races.

"Who wants to race?" I called out.

In less than a minute, both kids were on the floor with me, butts on an imaginary line, feet out straight.

"Get ready. Get set. Go!" I barked.

Off we went on a race that Mom always won. A race that gave the disadvantage to the people who had intact legs. We all sat on the floor with our legs extending in front of us. We made forward progress by lifting each butt cheek up and moving ahead a few inches at a time.

"It's not fair, Mom!" one of them said.

"My ankles get in the way," the other said.

"Waa, waa, waa" was always my response. "Aren't you jealous? See how lucky I am not to have legs?"

I never tired of playing this game, mainly because I always won. In fact, I've played it with lots of other people's kids over the years. It's the one thing many of them remind me of as they get older—how much fun they had butt-walk racing.

The kids may have lost that game, but it didn't take long for Tiffany and Brian to discover that they could take advantage of my disability.

"Enough!" I yelled for the umpteenth time. It had been a long afternoon, and the kids were at each other again. Teasing had turned into screaming and finally blows. I had to stop it before someone got hurt. But shouting "enough" had, if anything, only accelerated the feud. I jabbed the joystick on my wheelchair forward, trying to get close enough to administer a good smack to each child. Smart kids that they were, they took one look at me barreling toward them, spun around, and bounded up the stairs to a landing halfway up.

"Just you wait until your dad gets home," I sputtered.

"You can't get me, you can't get me" was their singsong taunt as they stared down at me.

"We'll see about that."

Totally frustrated, I turned my wheelchair and went back to the kitchen while they remained in the safety of the stairway landing. When Dave got home, I was waiting for him at the back door. Still annoyed, I told him about the afternoon debacle.

He barely put down his briefcase before calling out, "Tiffany. Brian. Get down here right now!"

They crept down the stairs and faced him.

"Tell me what happened today," he said.

Their mumbled answers were unsatisfactory. His reach was better than mine, and he spanked both of them.

"From now on, when your mom tells you to do something, you do it. If I ever come home again and hear that you ran away from her, I'll spank you twice as hard. Do you understand me?"

And so, for the rest of their childhood, if Mom needed to punish them, they made sure they stood right in front of me to get whatever was coming. They were probably the only children in the world who stood still to be spanked. While I know that spanking is frowned upon now, this incident reflects one of Dave's ironclad rules: it is crucial that parents support each other and present a unified front to their children. Parents are a team; they protect each other.

Dave took care of the financial affairs in our family, mainly because I was terrible at it and partly so I wouldn't have to worry about them. As soon as he arrived home each evening, he slit open the mail with a kitchen knife and methodically threw out the envelopes or placed the bills in their return envelopes awaiting the check for payment. He did this every single day at the same time, and I learned not to interrupt the process.

The necessity of building a wheelchair-accessible house had been a huge financial burden, in particular because of the sky-high interest rates in the early '80s. Our original construction loan had been 23.5 percent. When the house was done, Dave had refinanced a "take-out" loan that was a thirty-year mortgage on the house. We had to borrow $5,000 from each set of parents to have enough money in our bank account to qualify for the mortgage, which we got at about 18 percent. He refinanced our mortgage four times over the next three or four years to get the interest rate down to something manageable. Years later, he told me that he would often park on the street across from our house and sit there for a while, wondering how long we'd be able to live there because he didn't know if we had enough money to keep things going. He said he'd seriously considered taking a moonlighting job or taking out a type of loan from the Navy, known as a dead-horse loan, where they would advance you six months' salary.

"Have you seen the last bank statement?" Dave asked one evening after supper.

"No," I snapped at him. "I have no idea where you put it."

"Well, I need to balance the checkbook tonight, and I can't find anything in all these shit piles. It'd be really helpful if you'd at least *try* to stay organized," he said.

"Stop yelling at me," I barked, and it went downhill from there.

After five minutes of yelling at each other, I started crying. Dave kept ranting.

Finally, I couldn't take it any longer. I turned around in my electric wheelchair, accelerated, and ran right into him. He managed to move just enough that I didn't knock him down.

I couldn't believe what I'd just done. I was mortified. In all the years since the accident, Dave had never lifted a finger against me. Sure, there'd been lots of yelling, but he'd never hit me or abandoned me. Even when he was "seeing red," he always helped me put my legs on, pushed my wheelchair, helped me do whatever needed doing. I couldn't believe I was the one to have finally cracked.

In spite of appearances, we were like most couples in a lot of ways. We struggled and fought over all the same things "normal" couples fight over: money and sex and kids.

"It's been weeks since we've had sex" was the way it would usually start.

"What do you mean?" I'd retort, my heart beating rapidly because I didn't want to have this conversation. "What about last weekend?"

"What about it? I had to beg you to do it. I'm tired of always being the one to ask. Why can't you start it for once?"

I knew what he was saying was probably true, but I didn't want to admit it. I was constantly exhausted, and at times sex was just another chore, not the romantic interlude it had always been before children, jobs, and running a household.

It was probably the typical midthirties-married-couple dilemma, but at that time in my life, I felt an underlying current of fear. My body wasn't what it used to be, and I wondered if I would be able to continue to attract Dave. The combination of those fears and his frustration usually ended with my crying and telling him it wasn't his fault. Within the next few nights, I'd put on my sexiest lingerie, hoping that would be a signal that I'd heard him, that I understood, and that, deep down, I was still his Olsie and he was still the only man I wanted.

Our sex life wasn't of interest to only Dave and me.

"Mom," Tiffany said one day, "one of my friends asked me how you and Dad have sex."

"Yeah? And what did you tell her?"

She shrugged her shoulders and said, "'The same way as your parents, I guess.'"

Sex is something every kid wants to know and talk about until the subject comes around to their own parents. In my mind, I pictured Tiffany cocking her head and sarcastically adding, "I've never asked" or "I'm not watching."

If it was hard for our kids' friends to believe we had sex, it was even harder for some of their parents to imagine that I could exist at all.

One afternoon, the elementary school principal sought me out as I was picking up Tiffany and Brian from school.

"You aren't going to believe what happened yesterday," she said.

With a huge grin on her face, she continued, "RJ's mom marched into the office, demanding to see me immediately. She said, 'Tiffany Hodgens is going around telling lies. You need to make her stop! She's upset RJ so much that he can't sleep at night.' I innocently asked her what she could possibly be talking about." She flashed an impish smile and said, "I knew what was coming but couldn't help myself."

"So, what did she say?" I asked.

"She said, 'She's going around telling everyone that her mom doesn't have legs and an arm. You know that's impossible! You need to stop her from telling these outlandish stories.' I looked at her and asked, 'Have you ever met Tiffany's mom?' She said no, so I said, 'Well, maybe we should introduce you to her. Her name is Linda. She lost both her legs and her right arm before Tiffany and Brian were born. She's a doctor at UCSD. I'm sure you've seen her around; you just didn't realize it because when she's out and about, even though she walks with a cane and has only one arm, she looks and acts pretty much like you and me.'"

CHAPTER 10:

Get Out and Go!

....

"Hey, Linda, when you gonna get your butt back outdoors and go camping? You raising city slickers or real kids?" Carla taunted on the other end of the phone line. I was thrilled to hear her voice.

If anyone knew what it was like to be a city slicker, it was Carla. Seventeen years earlier, I'd been the one to introduce her—buttoned-up and always color coordinated—to the great outdoors when I'd invited her to climb Mount Whitney with me one summer when I was in med school. She'd quickly traded her penny loafers for hiking boots and has since climbed Kilimanjaro, Denali, and the tallest mountains in all fifty US states.

"How about canoeing the south end of Yellowstone Lake with us this summer? It's off limits to boats with motors, and there aren't any trails, either, so we'll probably have the place to ourselves!"

Her enthusiasm was contagious. Until I got off the phone. For minutes after I hung up, I sat motionless in the silence of the kitchen, staring off into space.

Many things disappeared from my life after the accident: playing the piano and pipe organ, riding my racing bike, swimming, and skiing. But what I missed most was being in the mountains. No more hiking or wilderness camping. Never again twirling around on the top of a mountain with my arms stretched to heaven. No more unlacing my hiking boots, pulling off heavy wool socks, and squealing as I gingerly dipped my feet in the icy snowmelt of a rocky mountain stream.

In the stillness, I was afraid. Truly afraid of being out there and knowing I couldn't experience it the way I wanted to—I, whose teenage dream was to spend her honeymoon backpacking all 211 miles of the John Muir Trail.

I was afraid to go to the mountains. I just knew it would make me think of growing up in Redlands, California. I used to drive up to the San Bernardino Mountains every weekend by myself. I'd get in my little Cortina and go up for two or three hours on Saturdays. Often, I'd just take a book. Now, I was afraid that the smell of the campfire, the smell of pine trees, the smell of water and rain would only depress me.

And be in the wilderness? Have the place to ourselves? Can we do this? Will I be a burden to everyone and ruin it for them? What if the kids hate it? What if Dave and Roger can't get along for four days?

Living in Montana and doing all the things she was doing, Carla was living my dream life. I envied her and her family's outdoorsy lifestyle.

I looked down and shifted in my chair. *No-legs Linda. In the woods. I don't know.*

But maybe it's time for it not to be just about me. I want our kids to experience rugged outback adventures and the risk-taking that goes along with that, not have a watered-down, namby-pamby, pretend-to-camp trip. Car camping in state-run campgrounds with Dave's parents in a pull-in spot next to wheelchair-accessible bathrooms wasn't cutting it. Maybe it was time to show the kids what I loved and to see the mountains again through their young eyes. Maybe watching them experience it would be enough to keep me from getting down.

Dave and I lay in bed and talked for hours that night. Well, mostly I talked. The gentle tingle of his touch as his fingertips caressed my shoulder and ran up and down my back told me he was listening.

"This could make us normal—beyond normal. It could give us the kind of life that I've always wanted to have."

"If you're ready, Olsie, let's go and do it." And, pulling me closer, he said what he says to me every night before he drifts off to sleep: "I can't live without you."

I have to do this. It's time, because this is what you do with kids. And if we don't, if I hold everybody back, our children will never get to experience the thing that I loved most in life.

A few days later, I decided that I was finally ready: ready to sleep under the stars on the hard ground in a little tent with the sighing sound of wind in the treetops lulling me to sleep, ready to smell the vanilla aroma of Jeffrey pines, and more than ready to smell like a campfire. When I was younger, I used to stash my dirty camping clothes in the back of my closet so I could enjoy the aroma of *parfum de campfire* for as long as possible.

My anticipation about returning to the wilderness was more than enough to allay my fear of depression. Nearly ten years after the accident and a week after her invitation, I returned Carla's fateful phone call. "Let's do it," I said. "I'm ready to get out and go!"

Of course, emotional readiness is one thing; practical readiness is another.

How does a severely disabled person get around without a wheelchair, go to the bathroom, and not add inordinately to everyone's work—and, and, and? All I knew for sure was that I could butt-walk and was small enough that I could be carried. The rest was a crapshoot.

~

The next few months were a whirlwind of planning: three canoes, four adults, four kids, four days, and twelve meals.

"I'm concerned about space," I told Carla. "How are we going to get all this stuff, *including food*, to fit into our canoes? What if we don't bring enough? It's not like we can call for takeout."

"Don't worry about it, Linda. I calculated the body weight and activity levels of all of us and counted calories to ensure we'll all have the appropriate number at each meal."

"Camping with a dietician—I should have known you'd have a plan."

"The thing is, the plan depends on our catching five or six fish every day, or we'll go hungry," said Carla.

"Great. Nothing like learning to hunt and gather under pressure. Dietician or not, we'll need lots of M&M's. No camping trip would be complete without 'em—and if Tiff and Brian end up hating camping, we can use the candy as a bribery tool!" Funny images of training puppies with treats flashed in my mind, but instead of fuzzy, eager animal faces, I saw the faces of my children. I couldn't help but giggle.

"Right," Carla replied.

"Okay, I think we've got the food covered, but this still feels pretty ambitious. We've never done this with kids, and it's not like I'm going to be able to paddle, Carla. What are we going to do about—"

"Linda, it's going to be fine. You'll be with us. Not only

will I make sure you don't starve to death, but Roger and I will
be right there with you. I promise. Nothing bad will happen
. . . but get life vests."

Life vests. Got it.

"Hey, hon," I said as I rolled into the living room, where
Dave was drinking a glass of wine and bent over a pad of
paper, "make sure to add life vests to your list."

"Already on there. Since you're here, come over here for
a minute. Let's go over this: TP, toothpaste, shampoo, floss,
liquid soap, cards, fishing licenses, airline tickets, money, maps,
camera and film, batteries, water bottles, compass, matches,
flint, pans, dishes and utensils, cups, washcloth and towel,
rope, trash bags, tent, dry bags, port-a-potty, shovel, flashlights,
knives, tarp, stove, water filter, *life jackets*, paddles, knee pads,
fishing gear, flares, whistle, binoculars. What am I forgetting?"

"I was thinking about what I'm going to wear," I said.

"Funny, I was thinking about you not wearing anything,
mountain mama." Dave flashed a charming smile, then got
back to the business at hand: "All right. When you *are* wearing
clothes, what are you thinking?"

"I'm thinking that I won't be able to wear my legs all the
time. So when I butt-walk, I'm going to need something that
keeps the dirt and rocks out of my delicate parts."

Dave took a sip of wine and raised his eyebrows. I continued, "Yeah, so I'll tie knots in the legs of a pair of jeans.
That'll protect my skin and keep the dirt out. And denim is
sturdy and won't show dirt. In fact, add extra pairs of jeans
for everyone to that list. And Carla mentioned rain gear, but
I don't think we need it, do you?"

"I hadn't thought about that yet."

"Well, I say we forgo spending lots of money on that
until we know whether we'll ever go camping again. I've never
carried rain gear in California and haven't ever needed it. Why
spend money on rain jackets when we can pull a few large trash

bags off a roll, make a neck hole in the bottom, and pull them over us on the off chance that it does rain? They also take up very little space in a stuff sack. Win-win situation."

"Sounds good to me. That's one less thing to buy."

Six months later, in August 1989, we flew to Missoula, Montana, where we packed two cars with camping gear and food and started driving to Yellowstone Lake. Carla and I had spent hours on the phone, planning the details and catching up with each other. I was excited about seeing her but still nervous about how the kids and men would get along.

The guy car started out in the lead, with the biggest canoe tied to its top. Carla and I followed, with two canoes strapped on ours. Before we knew it, the two giggly, wiggly, eight-year-old girls in the back seat had become best friends. With the windows down and the hot, dry air whipping our hair, Carla drove while I read through the flapping, handwritten lists of food and equipment, hoping we had everything we needed before it was too late to buy extra stuff.

"Mom, can we have more snacks?" Heidi asked.

"Yes, but no more M&M's, young lady. Eat some dried fruit. And share with Tiffany."

"Looks to me like they're arguing. What do you think?" I asked, squinting through the bug-splattered windshield at the car ahead of us.

For several miles, Dave and Roger had been waving their arms a lot. They kept jerking their heads back and forth. My stomach sank as I watched my fear play out before us. Carla and I put on our let's-be-happy faces as they pulled onto the shoulder of the road and got out. But before we could get our doors all the way open, we heard laughter—the loud, gut-rolling, har-de-har-har, guy kind of laughter.

The men needed a pee break, and so did I.

"All right, everyone. Eyes forward," Dave commanded as we positioned ourselves at the rear on the passenger side of the girl car. Pretending privacy, we slid my jeans and underpants down my stiff, metal-kneed prosthetic legs and, with my back to his front, we situated ourselves the only way I'd been able to figure out for a woman with two above-knee prostheses. Dave's big, strong, confidence-inspiring hands wrapped around my shoulders and arm. Legs extended in front of me, I leaned into him. The pressure of his hands on my skin increased as he took more and more of my weight. We shifted our weight and angles to accommodate each other in this lever-like maneuver that had Dave squatting and me in a wide-legged stance. All that to get into a good position to pee. *Knees. I really miss my knees.*

"All right. I'm done. Thanks."

"Okay. Up we go," he said, lifting us both with his legs and allowing me to pull myself together.

"Ooh, those look good. Share with your dad," Dave said, reaching into the backseat window and grabbing a handful of apricots from Tiffany.

Dave trotted off to Roger's car, I scrambled back into Carla's, and both vehicles pulled back onto the road.

A few minutes later, Tiffany called from the back seat, "Hey, Mom, I need to go to the bathroom."

"I'll take her," Carla said, pulling onto the shoulder once again.

Halfway out of the car, Tiffany started to cry. "I don't know how, Mom."

"Carla will teach you. It's easy."

Tiffany had never seen a woman with two normal legs squat to pee, but at eight, and before we even reached the lake, she had it wired.

The next morning, we sat through the mandatory park service lecture at Grant Village and learned how utterly stupid we must have been even to think about doing this trip. We solemnly confirmed to the park ranger that we'd read the following warnings:

- Canoeing and kayaking on Yellowstone Lake is a memorable experience, but it is not without its dangers. The water temperature, even in the summer, is typically forty to fifty degrees Fahrenheit. Almost daily, sudden winds create waves as high as four to five feet. These waves are choppy and very close together, making conditions especially hazardous for small boats.
- Travel close to shore and within sight of other party members. Begin early in the morning and avoid open-water crossings.
- Get off the water during strong winds and lightning storms.
- Practice capsize-recovery techniques with all party members prior to your trip.

The ranger scrutinized our three able-bodied adults, four young children, and woman missing both legs and one arm and shook his head.

Roger leaned in, put on his Marine face, and said, "Sir, we'll take good care of them." Carla, with her buff arms and legs sticking out of her T-shirt sleeves and shorts, backed him up with a hearty nod and promised to have us back in four days. I tried to keep a poker face in spite of the fact that if I had had knees, they'd have been knocking. I concentrated on suppressing all thoughts of the forty-plus people who'd drowned or died from hypothermia in this breathtakingly beautiful lake.

Corralling the kids, we got them to lug the waterproof bags, camp box, and ice chest onto the sandy beach. The over-size bags held forty to fifty pounds of food, four tents, eight sleeping bags, and our kitchen. Carla and Roger carefully positioned them in each canoe so we were balanced.

Leif and Heidi grasped the wood-rail edge of Carla's canoe and stepped in lithely. They'd clearly done this hundreds of times. Leif settled down on the front thwart. At age twelve, he was a blond, muscle-bound boy who was already stronger than his mom. Heidi took her place in the middle of their canoe, her perpetual, goofy smile and pigtails making her appear not to have a care in the world.

Even though I'd been an amputee for almost ten years, I still thought it crucial that I "look normal," so I wore my artificial legs with jeans and tennis shoes. After all the gear was settled and as Carla and kids pushed off from shore, Dave picked me up and carried all one hundred pounds of Linda and legs across the sandy beach, waded into the fifty-degree water, and slung me into the canoe, careful not to tip it over.

"Come on, kid. Can't get anywhere just standing there," Roger barked as he grabbed Brian and scuffled with him. In his early forties, Roger had thick, prematurely gray hair that belied his well-defined muscles and tan athleticism. The Marlboro Man without a cigarette, he'd have liked nothing better than to spend his life in the wilderness, sleeping on the ground and foraging for his existence. But he had a family, a PhD in forestry economics, and a job waiting for him at the end of this trip. We put all our trust in his outdoor prowess.

Since Roger's canoe was the largest and most stable, Brian got in with him. Five years old, Brian was only about thirty-five pounds and three feet, six inches tall and just fit on the tiny, weathered, wood folding chair that was part of the Cox family canoeing tradition. No-legs-no-arm Linda had been plopped on the floor in the middle of his canoe, fake legs sticking straight out in front of her, visible from the waist up, a position from which she could be seen and heard but could not serve any other useful function. It didn't take long before I felt the chill of the frigid water through the thin floor of the boat.

Tiffany climbed in unceremoniously and perched tentatively on the thin wood-slat seat in the front of Dave's canoe, her stringy white-blond hair squished under a pink baseball cap. Her white T-shirt was already dingy and her blue jeans wet from wading into the lake. She and Brian were both decked out in cheap bright orange life jackets with black nylon-webbed waistbands and a flat neck support pad that rested on their shoulders. Brian was so small that we had sewn a crotch strap on his so he wouldn't slide out of it if he went overboard.

"What are we waiting for? Let's get moving!" Roger barked in his drill sergeant voice. As soon as we were out of sight of the rangers, we threw to the wind our stay-along-the-shore promise and headed straight out across West Thumb Bay's five miles of open water. Neither Tiffany nor Dave had ever been in a canoe. Dave settled stiffly on the back seat and grimaced, his tightly clenched knuckles threatening to crush the paddles in his hands.

There was one major problem with this early morning scenario: Dave's canoe seemed to be defective. While Roger and Carla's plowed straight ahead, Dave's went left for a few feet and then swung right for a few feet, over and over again, zigzagging across the lake. The ten miles Carla and Roger paddled that day must have translated into twenty for Dave. *He's going to be exhausted. Gotta pull my weight, gotta be useful, gotta make this happen. . . .*

I began to sing, "Row, row, row your boat, gently down the stream . . ." Brian and Roger joined in. Our voices filled the gap between the canoes, and soon we were all singing our way across the lake.

Within ten minutes, a gust of wind whisked Brian's baseball cap off his head and sent it skittering across the water. Instinctively, he lunged for it. The boat rocked and tipped precariously. "Brian!" I yelled. "Sit down and hang on!" He grabbed the thwart in front of him with both his little hands, squeezed his eyes shut, and clenched his jaw, trying hard not to cry. The canoe tipped rapidly from side to side. My heart beat wildly. Visions of the last moments of other adventurers' lives blended with the reality of this moment: bodies in motion, no time to snatch a breath, the shock of cold, faces and hands above, the glint of sunlight through water, the press of empty lungs before a frantic grab for the surface, then a lifeless sink three hundred feet to the depths below.

We would not share that fate. Roger, ever the consummate guide, steadied our craft and coolly paddled on.

Breeze Point, Wolf Point, Snipe Point. Names on the map now had sandy or rocky beaches, evergreen trees, wildflowers, and a different vista as we rounded each craggy outcropping. I breathed deeply and opened my eyes wide—the eyes that led to my heart. Memory's knife slid down my chest and opened it to embrace the vistas and aromas, ensuring that they became part of my body and soul again.

Brian eventually rested his tiny body against mine. I stroked his soft hair as we slid through the landscape. My relaxation was complete. After all, we were in the middle of an enormous prehistoric caldera with densely packed forests of ancient lodgepole pines lining the lakeshore. Volcanic mountains shaped the horizon miles away. Bald eagles and ospreys swooped in and out of the trees, dive-bombing into the lake, and soared back up with fish in their talons. *What a majestic place.*

Way off over the mountains, puffy white clouds painted the quintessential Yellowstone postcard. Unnoticed by me, the shimmering surface of the lake had come to life. Rolling wavelets had started to wear frothy caps. And then, in less than ten minutes, the fabled Big Sky morphed into huge, roiling thunderheads climbing on top of each other and pushing a vicious wind across the water. My jaw dropped as I watched the storm line race toward us, pushing three-to-four-foot waves directly at us.

Roger and Carla brought their canoes closer together. Roger had saved us once, but he had his family to look after now. My stomach flip-flopped as I looked from canoe to canoe before locking on to Dave. How was he going to save us—a five-year-old who couldn't swim, an eight-year-old who thought she could do anything, and a wife with one arm?

A few big raindrops plopped onto my jeans and splattered my glasses. Within thirty seconds, I was soaked and watching water drip off Brian's nose and chin. In less than five minutes, I was floating in my own little lake in the bottom of the canoe. I looked behind me and saw Tiffany and Dave, heads bent low, squinting to keep the deluge out of their eyes so they could keep paddling.

I looked sheepishly at my family, all decked out in their jeans and T-shirts, and my heart sank. Suddenly, my vision of denim being a sturdy, durable fabric that wouldn't show dirt felt like a stupid, naive choice.

"I'm soaked," Brian groaned as he pawed through his dry bag. I dragged another bag through the water on the floor of the canoe while trying to untie the drawstring with my teeth and one hand. Rummaging through the tightly packed contents, I grabbed the first thing that felt like plastic, and out it came—a beautiful, large, white, very chic trash bag.

"Here, Brian. Put this on." His five-year-old look said, *And just how, Mom, does one put on a trash bag?* Oops. I grabbed it back, pulled it open, and sat there looking at it. What had I been thinking three weeks earlier? Oh, yes, tear a hole in the bottom so you can pull it over your head. *Why didn't I do that before we left home, when everything was nice and dry?* Turning the bag upside down, I grasped it with my teeth, ripped open a hole in the seam about the size of Brian's head, and handed it back to him. He obediently pulled it on and turned around to look at me. Everyone burst out laughing at the tousled, blond-haired head sitting atop a white bag. No-arms-no-legs Brian—just the comic relief we needed.

Pulling mightily with each stroke, Roger, Carla, and eventually Dave powered through the waves and paddled our canoes up to a narrow, isolated beach on the waves of a summer storm. There were no other boats on the lake, and there did not appear to be any campers at this end. The remoteness and water sloshing into the boats gave us a sense of urgency. Dave, Roger, and Carla landed their vessels. Roger snatched Brian up and out, and Dave hauled me out onto the wet, narrow, sandy beach and levered me down onto the ground.

I *looked* pretty normal but was inert on the packed black sand, with my fake legs, nice blue jeans, and shoes sticking straight out in front of me.

Behind me, Dave followed Carla and Roger's lead and dragged his canoe up to the tree line, where they all started feverishly unloading the bags.

Twisting around, I looked at the edge of what used to be a pristine forest but was now a charred black landscape covered by a layer of ash. There were tall black poles with snags, indescribably different from the green boughs on the Christmas tree–shaped pines in untouched portions of the park. In the short year since the massive Yellowstone fires of 1988, the decimated two-hundred-plus-year-old trees already had a bright green carpet growing under them. As my eyes focused, I saw an exotic spray of vibrant color from delicate, early wildflowers.

I needed to get out of those legs and into butt-walking mode. Above-knee prostheses are essentially replicas of the stilts from which clowns tower over us at the circus, and I'd be willing to bet that clowns walk only on very flat surfaces and in very wide-open spaces. And yes, my stilts technically did have knees, but they were unnatural contraptions that with the slightest misstep could send me crashing to the ground. I needed to get them off and under cover as quickly as possible. Not only were they all show and no go in this environment, they'd rust if I didn't keep them dry. I pulled myself over to my bag to retrieve my camp pants while everyone else buzzed around me.

"Hurry and get the tents up first, and make sure the rain flies are on them!" Roger directed. "Then get the food and kitchen stuff under tarps until this storm passes."

Ignoring us, the kids raced back down the beach, leaving a trail of wet clothes strewn haphazardly behind them. Their screeching and squealing reached us as they splashed into the lake to body-surf the storm waves in water the temperature of which the park ranger had warned us could lead to hypothermia in fifteen to twenty minutes. *Guess they missed that part of the lecture.*

Within an hour of our coming ashore, the lake was a sheet of silver-blue glass mirroring a huge crystal-blue dome overhead, and we started drying out. The M&M's and dried fruit had taken us as far as they could. Dinner was uppermost on our minds. Unless we got our butts in gear, set up fishing poles, and got back out on the lake, we'd be eight campers grumping around with growling stomachs. So Dave and Roger each retreated to a comfy rock and opened their sacred tackle boxes.

Dave sat up straight; glanced around; pulled out beautiful, shiny, bright red metal lures shaped like little fish; and started tying them onto spools of various colored lead-core line for us. Roger thumbed through his impressive array of dry and wet flies before choosing some woolly boogers that he tied lovingly onto four fly-fishing rods for his family. The men watched each other surreptitiously, the unspoken message between them being that fly fishing is beautiful and classy and trolling with lures, plebeian.

Well, we're going to need water. It was immediately obvious to me that this was a made-for-Linda job. I rummaged through the bags, found what I was looking for, and started to formulate a plan.

I cradled the pump and Nalgene bottles in my left arm and set off in my inimitable butt-walk to the shore. Goose bumps covered my arm. More than anything, I looked forward to the warmth and smell of our first campfire. Thrusting one hip forward and then the other, I made my way to the shoreline, happy for the knots at the ends of my camp pants that prevented the chilly wind from blowing up through the leg holes and pebbles from embedding themselves in my flesh.

I found a set of not-too-round, not-too-flat, partially submerged rocks, scooted into one, and grabbed a Nalgene bottle. It fit snugly between my legs, making it easier for me to unscrew its top. Tubing and filter in, I slipped the other end of the hose into the clear waters of the lake, allowing it to sink away from me.

We'd already had one hair-raising experience on the lake; the last thing we needed was giardia and cryptosporidium from the water ruining our trip. I wasn't keen on the idea of any of us contracting anything that could cause vomiting, diarrhea, or excessive gas.

While everyone else focused on getting fish, I watched Tiffany and Brian make the easy transition from city slickers to camp kids and started pumping. It was going to take a while, but I didn't care. I was doing something important—pulling my weight and being useful.

"Come on, kids. Let's get going." Dave steadied the canoe as he proudly handed Tiffany and Brian their fishing poles. Roger and Carla tried not to snicker as our city kids climbed into their dad's canoe, let out their lines, and started trolling away from shore. The Cox boats launched, and soon the fish-for-your-supper derby was in full swing.

After filling the bottles, I gathered the pump and tubing and butt-walked back to camp, leaving a line of closely spaced Vs in the sand. *It would be hard for me to get lost. Deer, elk, wolves, and bears leave tracks all over the park. Wonder what biologists would think if they saw this.*

"Fish on!" Dave shouted. The zing of a reel as the first fish made its run was proof. "Reel it in! Faster! Don't let the tip down," Dave instructed. It was a rapid-fire lesson on how to land this all-important prize. "Come on. Keep tension on that line!" He grabbed the fish net and deftly swooped a big Yellowstone cutthroat trout into the boat. The kids squealed and laughed, not knowing quite what to do with themselves or with the big fish that flopped out of the net and onto the floor. Dave quickly threw their lines back in, and the story repeated itself not once but several times.

Leif and Heidi watched jealously.

"Dad, can we use what they're using?" Leif asked. Roger adjusted his baseball cap and muttered something the still air didn't carry all the way to me.

When Dave and our kids had netted six or seven, they headed for shore to clean the fish and set up the campfire for cooking them, leaving our friends and guides looking bemused as they gracefully flicked their wrists and rods back and forward, in an equally successful choreographed dance of fishing.

As they approached, I called out, "Hey, kids. Grab those water bottles I left on the beach and bring them up with you."

After dinner, Dave dutifully gathered all the dirty dishes, along with camp suds, a washcloth, and a Teflon scrubber, and carried them to a secluded section of beach. From another spot closer to camp, I sat refilling water bottles.

There was no noise—no radio, no TV, no motors, no neighbors. Dave sat scrubbing dishes and gazing across the huge expanse of steel-blue water at the receding mountain ranges as the alpenglow faded and darkness enveloped the dense forest. The ground was cold under my jeans, and goose bumps crept up my torso, but I wasn't ready to leave.

Dave was a picture of peace. He is a man who immediately disables the dings, beeps, and chimes on every new appliance or gadget that enters our home and mutes the television when he watches sports; the quiet of the lake and forest suited him.

After a few minutes, sounds emerged from the silence— the faint splash of a fish jumping; the haunting tremolo and decrescendo of loons' evening conversations; the gentle lapping of wavelets on the shore; the scratching of the sand Dave was using to scrub the pots; and, somewhere behind me, the faint, occasional laugh of children playing Walk the Logs.

In the distance, ever the Marine, Roger summoned the troops in his drill sergeant voice: "Kiddos, over here!" When they had gathered in front of him, he asked, "Who wants to be eaten by a bear tonight?" He looked around at the stunned faces. "No takers? Fine. Then help me hang the trash way up in this tree. Which one of you can get this rope over that high branch up there? Winner gets M&M's!"

For the next ten minutes, Roger officiated while the kids competed in a game of Bear Keep-Away. In the end, they all got as many M&M's as their little fists could hold.

There were no losers that night.

Sitting there, I felt like I used to feel when we had a full moon in Redlands, where I could smell the orange blossoms and watch the moon rise over the mountains. It would be such a big, huge moon. It would look as if it were going to roll over the mountains. I used to have this feeling that I could just unzip my chest and that great big moon would come in, and the mountains would come in, and the orange blossoms would come in.

That was how I felt on the shores of Yellowstone Lake that night. I smelled the trees, and I could see that lake out there. I took a deep breath, pulling in as much of it as I could. *This is it.*

The shroud of night was black all around, and there were billions of tiny lights in the sky above. Our tent glowed faintly, lit from inside by squiggles from headlamps. Muffled giggles wafted through the flimsy tent walls as the kids tussled in sleeping bags, exuberant and exhausted.

Crouched in the doorway, Dave took one last look around camp before crawling into our tent and flopping onto his sleeping bag beside me. "My arms are going to fall off," he whispered. "We are coming back." And then he was asleep.

~

I wish I could say that I became instantly wise and relegated my fake legs to a waterproof bag for the rest of the trip, but I must confess that my pride still got the better of me. Every morning I made Dave help me get my legs on, lever up, and, while clutching his arm with a viselike grip, stumble down to the water's edge, where he would manfully sweep me off my feet and fling me into the canoe, in which I would pretend to be the queen of the Nile for another day.

Landing at our campsite on day two was much the same as the first day, but with less wind, waves, and wetness. After Dave extricated me from the canoe and plopped me down on the beach, he, Roger, and Carla hauled out all the bags and started setting up camp. The kids, who ended up wearing their life vests nearly twenty-four seven, jumped out, eager for their next adventure.

"Last one to find an arrowhead is a rotten egg," Tiffany yelled. With that, all four of the kids plopped belly down on the soft sand. Mother turtles about to lay a clutch of eggs could have taken lessons from those kids.

"You're a rotten egg," Leif said, digging frantically.

"Someone *smells* like a rotten egg," Heidi yelled, screwing up her face, crossing her eyes, and laughing as though she was having the most fun any child had ever had.

"Yeah, who farted?" Tiffany asked, giggling and digging faster.

"Backseat thunder!" Brian yelled.

"Backseat thunder!" Leif echoed.

All of us adults broke out laughing. That's what we got for eating ten dried apricots at a time for days on end. At least it wasn't diarrhea.

While the kids played and the other adults set up the tents, I found the perfect place to construct our kitchen. There must be a word other than *kitchen* to describe where we cooked. *Mess* comes to mind. To our credit, we did try to be picky about the sites. We looked for a flat space under a canopy of trees and with a nice long log or two for seating.

I reached for one of the wooden boxes that held our food and cooking gear and started pulling out large heavy-duty trash bags full of the prepackaged meals Carla had meticulously put together. Inside were smaller white trash bags, indelible ink marking each with a day of the week. One by one, I unpacked them: "breakfast," "lunch," "dinner."

Our large ice chest sat off to one side, but within a few butt-walk paces. I moved back and forth across the kitchen, making sure everything was out and within easy reach. The top of the ice chest served as a compact table just big enough for a stack of aluminum plates, plastic cups, inexpensive eating utensils, and a roll of paper towels that was always falling into the dirt. Roger's homemade plywood box with hinged top was stocked with essentials: seasonings in tiny containers, cooking oil, knives sheathed in a cloth with slots, aluminum foil, two dented pans, a nondescript coffeepot, a tiny camp stove with fuel bottle, and a beat-up frying pan.

It looked organized. Sort of.

Peals of man-size laughter and the thumping of back slapping regularly interrupted the squeals of joy from the beach.

"I still can't get over that . . . what do you call it—a port-a-poop?" Roger said, ribbing Dave as Dave headed off to find a private, more remote place to set up the port-a-potty he'd engineered. By day two, I'd figured out that I could just butt-walk out of the tent to pee in the night. I just needed to find a place with a small, flat rock and the right slope. If I put my right leg on the rock, I could hold myself up and pee without getting wet. *Why couldn't I have been born a guy?*

"That's about the stupidest thing I've ever seen," Carla said, with a good-natured laugh. "Just dig a hole and go behind a rock!"

"Yeah, sure," I replied, laughing and rummaging through one of the boxes, looking for the stove. "Watch the one-armed, no-legged lady dig a hole and poop in it."

Carla headed toward me, grabbed a bag labeled "day 2 snack," and sat down on one of two rough logs opposite me in our pine needle–carpeted dining room. She popped a handful of fruit and nuts into her mouth and gave me a sideways smile. Suddenly, we were back in college and everything in my life was how it was supposed to be.

Except for the stove.

That tiny, wobbly one-burner stove. Its eleven ounces were easy to lift with one arm, but using it almost required eight. Three skinny aluminum legs spread out to provide a base, and three blade-thin arms extended on top for a pot to sit on. Set up, it was pretty flimsy looking. But once it produced a flame, I became a consummate water boiler and knighted myself superintendent of all matters related to boiling and stirring the pot.

Sitting in the dirt, I tore open a bag of prepackaged rice and dumped the contents into the water I'd lovingly pumped from the lake and brought to a boil. Then came the hard part: stirring very carefully, with one hand, an eight-inch-wide pot on a teensy-weensy burner that wanted to do nothing more than tip over and burn me and fling its contents—our supper—onto the dirt floor of my kitchen. *No five-second rule here. I've got this. Yay, I have a job.* I wasn't useless after all!

~

Every day was an adventure: warm afternoons, cool nights, tearing down and setting up camp, paddling, fishing, swimming, digging, log hopping, wrassling, campfires and campfire songs, backseat thunder, laughing—so much laughing—and so much gentle lapping of waves, stillness, and quiet space to think and feel and see.

~

Legs on, looking like a normal, able-bodied mom in my plane seat, kids conked out beside us, I looked over as Dave turned to me, pencil in one hand, notebook in the other, and said, "Okay . . . next time. Here's what I've got: Allen wrenches, hiking poles, four Therm-a-Rests, two tents, four sleeping bags, tarp, stoves, fuel, matches, water pump, two kayaks—"

"Kayaks? I can't paddle."

"I've got an idea," he said, before going right back to his list. "Three paddles, kettles, frying pans, water jugs, Ziplocs, backpack, boat shoes—two pairs—rain jackets and rain pants, blue foam pads, sunscreen, bug repellent, throw rope, anchor, dry waders, break-down paddle, long nylon pants, bilge pump, lightweight rain shelter, kayak dry sacks. That's my list. What's on yours?"

"Numbers one through ten are to figure out a better way to make my camp pants. Those knots have got to go! Next time, I'm going to take a pair of jeans and fold the legs up backward under me to make a three-layered butt pad. If we sew them all the way around, they'll be sturdy and will keep the dirt out. I love nature, but I don't think I need to be that intimate with it."

"Great idea. And I've got some ideas for how to improve our port-a-potty. They gave us a lot of crap about it, but did you notice that even the king and queen of the wilderness used it?" Dave asked. The corners of his mustache twitched upward, and he continued scribbling notes as the plane gently sped us home through the clear blue sky.

"Well, you couldn't beat the view from that throne," I replied. "Hey, since you've got your paper and pencil out, food for thought: less oil, but more teriyaki; soups; meats for lunch, like sausage and jerky; bagels; peanut butter; extra granola for snacks. Likes: tortellini; that jalapeño cornbread; regular cornbread; spicy couscous; and definitely more oatmeal, carrots, and hot chocolate."

The kids slept off the adventure behind us as I leaned against the airplane window. We'd done it. I'd butt-walked in the dirt, somehow managed to poop and pee in a semirespectable fashion, cooked on the pine-needled ground, filtered the water, and watched my family have the time of their lives. Dave and I continued to talk and scribble notes, energized by all the adventures we could now see in front of us.

CHAPTER 11:

Stopped, Dropped,
and Rolled with It

....

"I'm almost done. Be there in ten minutes," I promised as I hung up the phone in the pitch-black radiology reading room at UCSD's Thornton Hospital, where I'd been interpreting chest X-rays with the resident assigned to the service. It was August 27, 2007—twenty-eight years to the day since the accident. As soon as I finished dictating my last case, I planned to drive to the Breast Imaging Center for my afternoon shift of reading mammograms and breast ultrasounds.

It was a short walk down the hall to the double glass doors leading out of the hospital. I pushed the door open, took one step outside, wobbled for an instant on a wrinkle in the large doormat, and went down like a tree being felled. When I hit the sidewalk, an excruciating dagger of pain ripped through my body. It took all of five seconds to know that my hip was broken. It took five more seconds for someone to walk out the emergency room's door and notice me lying there, squinting up at the sky, fist clenched.

"Do you need help?"

The words floated somewhere over my head. This time, they were in English. This time, my legs were still attached. Of course I needed help. Even if my hip wasn't broken, when on the ground, my fake legs were as useless as my real ones had been as I'd lain on the tracks after the train hit me nearly three decades before.

"I need somebody to take me over to X-ray to see if I broke my hip."

"Hold on," the voice said. "I'll go get somebody from the ER."

Come on! Just get me back over to Radiology.

The voice moved away, calling for someone to come and help rescue me.

"Shit," I said to myself. I wiggled my left arm to confirm that at least my wrist was okay. An ER tech and nurse rushed out with a backboard, cajoled me to scoot over onto it, lifted it onto a gurney, and rolled me back into the emergency room.

Another August afternoon. Another accident. Another twist of fate.

- X-rays—check
- nondisplaced left hip fracture—check
- IV running and first dose of morphine—check

Within ten minutes, I was loopy but still with it enough to realize that this might change things. In twenty-six years, I'd missed only one week of work. Being disabled, I'd always worried about not pulling my weight. *Will I be able to work? More important, will I ever be able to walk again?*

That morning, I'd been perched in my wheelchair at home, artificial legs partway on, drumming my fingers on the counter near the back door, waiting for someone to kneel on the floor between my fake feet and strain to pull me down into the tight suction sockets of my prostheses.

For a moment, my mind flashed back to the days when I was pregnant with Tiffany and completing my residency in Los Angeles. I'd had Iron Mike, the device we called my best friend because without him I couldn't have lived by myself. Once I got my permanent suction-socket prosthetics, I'd never been able to put them on by myself. So, for twenty-six years, Dave or the kids, our parents, brothers, sisters, neighbors, nannies, housekeepers, and even strangers had had to perform this procedure for me. That morning, our neighbor Maria Bauz was on call. I'd have given anything to be able to do it by myself, anyplace, anytime.

"Hiya," she said. "Are you ready?"

I'd already powdered my legs and pulled the stockinet stockings all the way up to my groin. The other ends hung out through the valve holes at the bottoms of the sockets.

"Let's do it," I said as I pushed on the arm of my wheelchair and levered myself to a precarious upright position. She wrapped a stocking around her hand, leaned down, and tugged, slowly pulling my leg into one artificial leg. Her wrists and forearms slammed on the floor as the stocking emerged through the hole in the socket.

"Thanks," I said as she finished the second one. "I really appreciate you getting up early to come do this."

"No problem. Anytime." She flashed me a big grin, rolled her eyes, and pranced back home in her pajamas. *Wonder if she'd think it was a problem if she had to do that every day.*

My foggy brain floated back to the ER, where the nurse wanted me to undress and put on a hospital gown. Taking off my blouse was slow but doable. Removing my slacks was a different story.

Before I realized what was happening, she unzipped them and started tugging.

"Stop! You're going to pull my leg off!" I yelled. The nurse's pulling jarred my newly broken left hip. She looked at me as if I was crazy.

"Your leg isn't going to come off; it's just broken."

"Oh, yes, it will!" I screamed. "They're fake. Don't touch me." Her look this time said she thought I was completely nuts.

"Here," I said, grabbing her hand and pressing it on the top of my rigid prosthetic socket. Her eyes got big as she yanked it away.

"Well, we have to get them off somehow." Out she went for reinforcements. That turned out to be another nurse and a second dose of morphine. Oh my, that did the trick. Once the pants were off, they started talking about taking both my legs off.

"Nooo . . . we can't do that," I said, slurring only slightly. I was still lying on the backboard and by then had figured out that it would be to everyone's advantage for me to keep my legs on. Since they're suction sockets, it takes a lot of force to remove them—enough force that it would definitely have displaced my fracture and been excruciatingly painful. They were still shaking their heads as they left the room.

"Hey, Linda, how are you feeling?" asked my friend and fellow radiologist, Meg Richman. Word traveled fast, and my colleagues had started arriving in my room.

"Fine," I lied. It hurt like hell. Worse than the train accident. I fooled no one. At least they hadn't cut my pants off like the people in Salzburg had.

"Hey, does Dave know about this?" Mary O'Boyle was another friend and radiology colleague.

My tongue was now under the control of morphine, my speech more rapid and run-on.

"No, he's off hunting. I don't think we can reach him. I don't want to ruin his trip. Let's just not call. I don't want him to worry he has someone else with him and I don't know wheretheyarehe'llfindoutwhenhegetshomesometimenextweek. . . ." I stopped to take a breath.

Mary jumped in before I could start in again. "Come on, Linda. You gotta let him know!"

"Okay, okay. Hey, can you call him?" Her husband, Bill Keen, was actually the person Dave had been hunting with in a remote part of Canada. They were due home later that day. It was getting hard to make sense.

When Dave and Bill reached Chicago, they got the message that I was heading to the operating room for repair of a fractured hip. That evening, Mary met them at the airport in San Diego and offered to drop Dave at the hospital. He politely refused and headed home to take a shower and get the caribou into the freezer. There was nothing he could do, and he'd be at the hospital by 9:00 p.m., in time to see me come out of anesthesia. He'd be holding my hand and smiling at me when I woke up.

~

The day after surgery, the physical therapist assigned to me popped into my room.

"Hi. My name's Sarah. I'm here to teach you how to transfer from your bed into the wheelchair, make sure you can ambulate to the bathroom, and show you how to use crutches."

She stood next to my bed, a petite young girl with short, curly black hair. She smiled and leaned on the back handle of my wheelchair. She didn't seem to notice that the front of the wheelchair faced the bed and was pushed up against the edge of it so I could butt-walk into it.

"I'm going to show you how to stand up and transfer over into this wheelchair," she said as she unlocked the brakes and rolled the chair away from the bed.

What is she thinking? Is she blind?

I took hold of the sheet and, gritting my teeth, slowly pulled myself upright. Turning gingerly and supporting my bandaged leg with my left hand, I butt-walked to the edge of the bed, all the time watching Sarah's face.

"If you just put my wheelchair back where it was, I'll show you how I scoot over into it so I can go to the bathroom. It's a piece of cake. Didn't they tell you I don't have legs?"

"I, er, huh . . . Oh my God!" she gasped. "How do you do that? What happened to you? I feel so stupid. . . . How can I help?"

I don't need help. I don't want help. I just want to be back to my normal and back at work.

Five weeks later, dressed in khaki shorts and a nice blouse and without my prostheses on, I pushed my one-arm-drive wheelchair into work.

The first tech walked right past me. *That's strange. We say hi every day.* I sat up a little straighter as I rolled down the hall. *I'm back to looking at people's belly buttons. . . . I'd better start talking so they'll have to look at me.*

"Hi, Patrick. How are you?" I asked the next person coming toward me. He stopped abruptly and tilted his head as he peered down at me. I waited and smiled at him.

"Pardon . . ." And then he stopped. "Dr. Olson?" he said incredulously.

"Yup," I said. "It's me. I just don't have my legs on today."

"I've never seen you in a wheelchair. And . . . I've never seen you without legs!"

"I know; this is my usual after-hours attire," I said with a giggle.

"I'd heard you fell and broke your hip. . . ." And then he burst out laughing. "Don't you think that's carrying it a little

too far? Cutting off your legs just because you broke a hip?"
He couldn't contain himself. "What a great joke, Dr. Olson!"
I'd worked there for twenty-six years, but people were
always dumbfounded when they saw me for the first time as
a tiny little person without legs in a wheelchair. I'd told the
accident story a thousand times over the years; they all knew
what had happened. Even though I walked with a quad cane
and an awkward toy-soldier gait, most of them had never truly
understood what was really wrong.

Over the next few weeks, it became clear that the soft-tis-
sue shape of my left leg was different enough after the surgery
that I needed to have a new socket made. In the ten years since
my last legs had been fabricated, C-Legs, the first micropro-
cessor-controlled knees, had been invented, and silicone liners
had replaced the old method of donning with stockings and
powder. My prosthetist, Kevin Calvo, thought I'd be a good
candidate for this new technology. I was excited about the
prospect of becoming a modern, robotic woman.

To my dismay, the electronic knee experiment was a failure.
While they allowed me to sit down in a more ladylike fashion,
they caused problems. While I was driving, the lower part of the
leg would lift, taking my foot off the floor. And I was working
and didn't want to take time off to learn how to use them. After
a few weeks of struggle, I went back to the mechanical knees I'd
used so successfully for twenty-eight years.

The new silicone liners, however, were a life-changer.
At age fifty-eight, I experienced newfound independence that
I'd never dreamed I'd have again. The new technology allows
amputees to roll a silicone liner up over their residual limb—
like putting on a big gray condom. After those were on, with
the aid of a spritz of alcohol, I could slip in and out of the
suction sockets almost as easily as everyone else does their
shoes. I could motor my wheelchair up to my fake legs, which
waited in patient repose in the corner of our bedroom, scoot

into them, and in less than two minutes bring my legs to life. Another silver lining.

My fall and game-changing freedom were ironic and prophetic.

Broken hips are an old-lady ailment that often heralds a slow downhill slide, but my fall brought me greater freedom and hope. But I was now more aware than ever of Father Time and of the reality that although I'd successfully fought my way back to as close to normal as I could get, I really was mortal. I would become more limited as time went on. It was equal parts elation and frustration.

I became obsessed with the fear of falling and breaking another hip, so I started taking my manual wheelchair to work. I pushed it ahead of me like a walker as a means of increasing my stability. Just like when I'd started learning to walk, I simply put my head down and did it, pretending I didn't know or care about how funny it looked.

Reality finally sank in, and after I retired, I transitioned to a van with a lift in the back for an electric wheelchair. Back to belly-button height and craning my neck to look up at people talking to me. But, for the first time since the accident, I could independently get in my wheelchair and zoom five miles per hour, up and down a shopping mall or at the beach or around my neighborhood, several miles before needing a charge.

My clumsy stumble and broken hip allowed me to get out and go whenever and almost wherever I wanted. My schedule is no longer dependent on someone else's availability. I don't have to ask for help: no leg-puller sitting on the floor between my legs, trying not to look at my crotch. People don't need to arrange their day around mine. And, as important, it's one more thing that gives me independence and one less reason for Dave to worry about me.

~

"I'm ready," I said.

My college roommates, Juli and Carla, and I were in Livingston, Montana for our annual birthday celebration get-together.

It was a worn-out phrase they'd heard me say for almost twenty-nine years. But this time, no one sat down on the floor to pull off the stockings. This time they came in and leaned against the wall while I pushed myself out of my wheelchair and stood up.

"Can you believe this? I'm . . . " My voice wavered, and I couldn't speak. I wiped my eyes with my right sleeve. "I'm . . . putting . . . my legs on . . . by myself!"

Tears ran down our faces.

~

"Pardon me," I said to the man sitting beside me. Our plane was London bound, and we still had six hours to go. "I just want to give you a heads-up." He smiled pleasantly but didn't look up. "If you wake up in the middle of the night, half of me will be on the floor."

He turned, his full attention on me.

I grasped the jeans on my right thigh and pulled my leg up. "These are fake legs, and I plan on taking them off pretty soon. I'll just lay them on the floor. I don't want them to scare you." I flashed my big so-what-are-you-going-to-say grin and waited.

"Really! That's pretty cool!" he said. And, of course, then I had to tell him the story, the accident story, which over the years had turned into a love story.

"This is my daughter," I said, pointing at Tiffany, who was sitting beside me. "Both our kids were born after the accident, so this is the only way they've ever known me."

With tears in his eyes, he asked, "Do you mind if I tell my kids when I get home? They need to know your story."

~

By the time I was fifty-eight, I'd lost my right arm and both legs and broken a hip, but I was okay. More than okay. I'm okay whether I'm walking with protheses, whether I'm in a wheelchair, and whether I have my legs on or off.

The world is far more accessible than it once was for me, and I now have a lot of independence, but I'll always be somewhat dependent upon others. And that's okay, too.

Carry On

"I hate dependency." The thought of a strong-minded, independent young woman, one who had climbed Mount Whitney twice and was undaunted by a fifty-to-one-hundred-mile bike ride.

"I'm embarrassed to be seen being carried." The thought of every young woman or man concerned about how they fit into the world.

Linda, with mental strength beyond imagining, buried all this negativity and embraced our shared roles. The prospect of access to the places we loved— the beach, the mountains, the countryside—was enough for her to push all those feelings into a box from which they have never emerged.

Together, we advanced. I modified a pack frame, literally made for a hunter to carry a deer, so that I could carry my dear. And she adopted a spirit of gracious dependence. With a set of shoulder straps mounted in reverse, Linda could sit comfortably on the seat, safely buckled in by the straps, and ride on my back. When she was dressed in hiking clothes and carrying a liter of drinking water, the whole enchilada weighed about ninety pounds. A heavy pack, but doable.

I love this feeling of strength, of power, and of romance. But it goes way beyond that. She needs me. Going from point A to point B has become an exercise in intimacy between us and invisible to others. The carrying is part of our bond. It is also something that stirs and evokes something primitive and ancient in the soul of every man who sees us. I'm carrying my woman off. Off to wherever to do whatever. Every man wants to do this. Every man feels this instinctive need.

Years later, as we reveled in the wonders of Machu Picchu in Peru, I saw this confirmed again.

To tour Machu Picchu means to walk, to go up and down steep staircases of rock. After we stopped to rest, our guides offered to take turns. After the first guide's turn, I leaned in to take over. Jose, who was carrying Linda at the time, looked at me with a serious stare. I turned, and Washy was giving me the same look. It was Benjamin, our principal guide and the one whose turn it was next, who articulated their thoughts: "I will never get a chance to do this again in my life. Would you take this pleasure away from me?" They had discovered Linda. They had discovered the intimacy of carrying and of being carried.

"No, Benjamin," I said, returning his smile, "I will not take this experience away from you."

As he hoisted her up onto his back, a grinning, happy Linda looked over his shoulder at me. For now, she belonged to them.

"Yo lo comprendo," *I stammered back in rudimentary Spanish. I knew how he felt.*

I had seen that look before. In the eyes of the train porters and every hiker we'd encountered on trails across the Americas.

We could canoe, and we could do backcountry. The frame allowed me to carry Linda easily on the portages from lake to lake on long, wonderful circuits in Canada and the United States, where we camped and fished and let our kids have the run of a purely natural world for two weeks at a time. We occasionally saw other people who were pleasantly surprised by the two-headed voyageur coming toward them on the portage trail. Linda's grin and banter immediately disarmed them, and they went their way, having had their day biased toward the positive. I began to notice the look in the eyes of the men we encountered. They were jealous. I deserve to be envied.

CHAPTER 12:

Save Me!

....

A hot Santa Ana wind had been blowing all week, with gusts measuring up to one hundred miles per hour. Wildfire reports blared incessantly on our radio stations. Needing a distraction and thinking about writing a book, I asked Dave if he could look in our storage locker for any boxes that might have stuff from after the accident.

He returned home with an old Perma Pak storage box and left it in my office. It was late in the evening when I noticed it, faded black capital letters on each side spelling "MEMORABILIA." Inside was a clutter of tattered envelopes, tabbed manila folders, and a few notebooks that memorialized grade school, college, and beyond.

At the top of one folder, "Ovens & Stoves" was crossed off and "Salzburg" printed in black ink underneath. This was what I needed. I was on a mission to find things that would jog my memory of the immediate post-accident period. Three other folders looked promising, too: "Accident Documents," "Military Service Documents," and "Letters, Etc."

I couldn't recall ever having seen the accident file. As soon as I pulled the front of the "Accident Documents" open, I saw a folded piece of white paper:

Polizeiinspektion   8420 Berchtesgaden, 02.04.1980
Berchtesgaden
B-Tgb.Nr. 505/80
Frau
Linda Hodgens

Two paragraphs followed, all written in German and signed "Ernst, Polizeihauptkommissar."

Sixteen black-and-white photos were stacked neatly inside the folded paper, as if waiting to show me something—and waiting to see if I had the courage to look. I refolded the letter and sat motionless, staring at the large, dreamy watercolor of Salzburg that hangs on my office wall. Its lush shades of blue, green, and warm yellows drew my eyes across the Salzach River into the quaint streets of Old Town, with its steepled skyline, and up a steep hill to the ancient, walled Hohensalzburg Fortress. For years, this painting has personified serenity for me.

I slouched in my wheelchair with what was left of my legs propped against the desk for balance, put the photos on my lap, and thumbed through them halfheartedly. They had maintained their glossy finish and crisp blacks and whites as though they'd been taken yesterday.

The first photograph showed a railroad curving into the distance with a grassy bank that led down to a small river on the right. Beautiful forest trees lined this corridor. It could have been used in an art book as a good example of perspective.

The second offered a different kind of perspective. I was jolted by the scene reflected: a VW van askew on the tracks, tilting down at an angle, the front two wheels between the rails, the back two resting higher, on cement siding. An ambulance and fire truck were partially visible on the sides of the tracks and in the background. Again, a tall forest provided the backdrop. Picture three was a duplicate.

The next showed four small, numbered evidence marker signs extending into the distance. Something white lay on the rail bed. *Maybe a piece of clothing?* The van was off the tracks, near the trees along the right, its midsection bashed in.

Picture five showed more little signs. I could see tire drag marks in the dirt leading to the van, which had been pulled off the tracks and toward the trees.

Sign number one drew my attention. There was something in the dirt, but it was hard to see. I rolled over to a drawer and pulled out my magnifying glass, the one I'd used for more than thirty years when looking at mammograms.

It was a shoe. *Maybe a left shoe?* I laid down the lens for a minute and stared out the window into the blackness of the night, wondering if it was my shoe or Dave's. I took in a deep breath and looked again. There wasn't anything sticking up above the top of it, so I was pretty sure it belonged to Dave. One of my most vivid memories of the accident was seeing a shoe with my severed foot in it lying a few feet from me and then watching someone place it on the gurney with me as I was lifted into the ambulance. It looked so prim and proper with the shoelaces neatly tied.

The next three photos showed a brick road paved in a repeating scallop pattern with a railroad track crossing it, nothing else. Rather artistic for a mountain byway.

Number nine was a full-on side view of the crushed passenger door, with an ice chest visible inside the van. I suspected it had cheese and bread in it, the remainders of our afternoon picnic outside the city of Ulm.

I sat very still for a couple of minutes. *Should I go on? I lived this story thirty-five years ago. I'm happy. I've never had nightmares. Is there a chance these pictures will trigger something bad?*

With one finger, I touched the top of photo nine and pulled it forward to see what was next. Some kind of vertical, linty, white artifact gave this photograph a surreal appearance. The van was still angled sideways across the tracks and tilting down. But in this one, the front passenger door was hanging open, and there was a train engine twice the size of the van abutting the driver's side. An empty gurney with a white sheet and pillow was waiting on the ground. Several onlookers crowded the back left edge of the picture. The photograph was so still, yet charged with the emotion of something awful that had just happened but was already in the past.

And then number eleven, with a different angle of the engine looming behind the van. God, it was huge. A real-life monster looking straight at me with headlight eyes and a black grille grinning grimly across its lower half. Two men on their hands and knees were leaning over something right up against the van. A third, dressed in white, hovered over them. Their heads were bent low near the ground.

Again, I picked up the magnifying lens. Something was lying on the ground, barely visible between two of the men. I squinted and kept moving the magnifier up and down to focus as it dawned on me that they must be trying to talk to someone.

Is that me? I paused. *Maybe I should look at this in the morning.* But I couldn't. I couldn't wait.

I moved to a brightly lit corner of my office and circled the magnifying glass around the picture more thoughtfully, wondering who else I might recognize. A petite blond woman was talking to two men. Dave's mom. *Donna.* The man with his back toward the camera was Dave's brother. *Mark.* I suspected they were talking to the police. I had already read their official statements, which had been typed in German and English and were now yellowed by age. Photo eleven might portray the time when they were making their statements.

I looked once more at the figure on the ground and knew without a doubt that it was I. Slowly, I laid down the magnifying glass and reran the vivid thirty-five-year-old memory reel in my mind. It happened so fast. I'd always remembered the passengers rushing off the train, shouting to each other in German and then lifting up the van to pull me out from under it. Now, I saw it in these glossy black-and-white photos from outside myself, at a distance from the scene.

It's strange how this did not change the way I felt. I looked down at my armless shoulder and touched the ends of both my very short legs. This is who I am, a triple amputee with no right arm and both legs off above the knees. Even after sitting still for a few minutes, I had no tears.

I was going to die, but then I didn't.

And when I didn't, I grabbed on to the hope that I'd live.

I knew that if I did live, I could make it work.

And when Dave hobbled into the ICU the next day and said that he hadn't married my arms and my legs, that if I could do it, he could do it, I knew that we would make it work.

I knew that I must expend all the energy I could muster to keep Dave from being discouraged. My strength grew while I helped everyone around me see the possibility of a bright future. I wanted to keep laughing and to hear laughter around me. There was no time and not enough energy to spend on being morose, going to dark places, or asking, "Why?" and "What if?"

I gathered the pictures and tapped the edges to straighten them into a neat stack. The front picture showed a tranquil railroad curving into the distance with a grassy bank leading down to a small river on the right. It hid the rest. Sometimes hiding prevents us from moving forward. Sometimes it's the only way to move forward. Besides, it was a lifetime ago.

~

Brian had been staying with us, and it had been a long week. Everyone was tired. The muffled conversation between Dave and Brian coming from the kitchen got louder. I busied myself at the far end of the house, waiting for things to settle down, but the argument reached out to me.

"I'm thirty years old. Why can't she stop worrying about me?" Brian said.

I suspected it had something to do with my having told Dave how hard it was to get a good night's sleep when I kept waking up at night, waiting to hear Brian come home.

"Brian," Dave said, "you need to give your mom a break. I know she worries, but there are reasons for that!" The tone had shifted from father-son to man-to-man.

I started toward the kitchen but stopped when Dave proceeded, in a more measured tone: "I think it's time you know what really happened when we got hit by the train. It might help you understand your mom a little better."

I held my breath.

Brian said nothing.

Dave continued, "You know we were on vacation in Germany with my parents and Mark and his wife." He paused. "I don't know how to say this . . . but it's time you know that we didn't really *stall* on the railroad tracks."

He hesitated, then went on. "We were lost. We'd been driving up a narrow mountain road, trying to get to Berchtesgaden. There was no place to pull over, so when *my* dad, *your* grandfather, saw a flat stretch of road ahead, he decided to stop there so he could look at the map. He had just turned off the engine and reached for the map when your mom saw a train coming around the corner. She yelled for him to get off the tracks. . . . Then we all saw it. Everyone yelled, but he couldn't restart the engine." His voice cracked as he continued.

"It was a stupid mistake on my dad's part. He was stubborn and determined to look at that map. That decision cost your mom her legs and her arm and forever changed our lives."

I went a few feet farther down the hallway and stopped again, wondering what Brian's reaction would be. It was Dave who spoke. "A couple of nights after the accident, your mom told me she wanted to talk about what had happened. She told me she could remember everything: how my dad stopped the van so he could look at the map, how my dad and I and Mark got out of the car, how she fell out onto the tracks, how I picked her up. The train slamming into the van. When the train stopped, everyone got off and pulled the van off her. She never lost consciousness."

Brian said nothing.

"I listened and told her that was the way I remembered it, too. We talked and we cried. We talked about our families and how difficult it was for them to see her so terribly disabled, to think that our lives would never be the same again. And then we talked about our future. How we wanted to have children. How important it would be for our families to help us if we did. We were pretty sure it would tear our families apart if your mom's parents found out what had really happened. And we knew beyond a doubt that my dad would live with the guilt of his choice for the rest of his life."

I decided it was time to join the conversation; plus, I wanted to see how Brian was reacting to this news.

As I approached the door, Dave said, "So, we made a pact that night. Rather than tell our families—and everyone who knew us—that my dad stopped on the railroad track to read a map, we would tell them that our van *stalled* on the track."

They both turned toward me as I came into the kitchen and picked up where Dave had left off. "Even though it was only three days since the accident, I already knew that it was going to take every ounce of energy I had to learn how to walk, learn how to use my left hand, go back to work. I wanted to get that behind me as fast as possible. We both knew exactly what had happened. It would do us no good to spend time and energy on blame, what-ifs, or whys. What was done was done."

Brian stood quiet but not alarmed.

I continued, "One of the hardest things for me from day one was seeing how devastated our families were. I quickly realized that I was the only one who could make them feel better. That it was my job to get them to laugh and believe that we were going to be all right. This little white lie was the only way we knew to take back control of our lives. I wanted to be happy, and I wanted everyone around me to be happy, too. . . . And, most importantly, I wanted Dad to be happy so he'd stick around and not leave me."

Dave leaned over and hugged me. "Olsie, I'd never have left you," he said for the millionth time.

The room was silent. Dave stood next to the stove. Brian leaned on the kitchen counter. Silver-haired dad and the younger blond son. No one spoke. It was as if the words were working their way in and through our son's being. I could only imagine how it must feel to hear such a damning statement about his beloved grandfather.

And then Brian turned and said, "It's funny. It doesn't matter. We've had a wonderful life, and what's done is done."

～

Life was good, and the accident was part of the fabric of it. Our granddaughter, Sierra, has heard the train story many times and turned it into her own little reality show: Train Wreck. This reenactment played out in a vacation condo in Truckee, California, when she was five years old.

"Save me, Grandpa! Save me! Is this the way it was?" Sierra said while lying on the floor. We've played Train Wreck umpteen times, and each time, she carefully positions her body so she is parallel to the grout lines in the tile floor. Each time, Dave checks her position, makes a couple of adjustments, and then nods his approval.

"Okay, now save me!" she called.

Dutifully, Dave went to the other end of the room, turned around, and ran back across to her, shouting, "I'm here! I'm here!" He hooked his hands under her armpits, pulled her up, and hugged her to himself.

"Then what happened?" she asked. She knows, of course, but the telling and the doing, in every minute detail, are part of the game.

"Well, the train hit us and tore your grandmother out of my arms and pinned her to the track," he recounted while gently releasing her back to the floor, where she collapsed in a blond heap.

He continued, "And then, after it knocked me off to the side, it dragged her down the railbed"—a concept I'm not sure she grasps yet. Sierra lay in a heap on the "tracks," listening intently, eyes open and present.

"Did it hurt, Grandma?" she asked as she turned toward me.

No-Leg Grandma, as I'm called, is always sitting nearby when this game is being played, and I responded the same way I always do: "No, sweet face. I didn't feel any pain; I just felt my breath being squeezed out of me."

"Grandpa, save me!" Sierra called out again.

This is the part where Dr. Grandpa has to examine the limp body at his feet and check pulses, listen to breath sounds, open each eye and look at the pupils, and go through—without leaving out any detail—a finger-and-toe count before he can finally declare that she is in fine form, with no contusions, no fractures, and no residual effects from our pretend harrowing experience.

I watched the scene play out and on cue chimed in, "Make sure she still has tickle spots that work," which served to reanimate the flaccid five-year-old, who sprang up, laughing and squealing, before running out of the room.

"Okay, Grandpa—your turn! I'll save you!"

As was expected, Dave slowly got down on the floor, spread out supine, and got his body and limbs in just the right position so she could run across the room and pick him up off the tracks.

They've exchanged roles. She will never know how many times her grandfather has wished that he could have done just that on an August afternoon in Bavaria.

Later that day, Sierra called out to me this time, "It's almost time to go!"

It was time to get the skis out, and our adventuresome, impatient, bubbly little granddaughter looked at me and said, "Get your legs on, Grandma!"

CHAPTER 13:

Eighty Thousand Miles

··

O-dark-thirty. Out the door he went in his old, faded cotton shirt with its stretched-out neck, white tube socks, low-top Converse All-Star shoes, and baggy white shorts. Starting at a slow trot with measured breathing, he leaned forward and gradually picked up the pace. He had miles to go.

I noticed him the first day of medical school. Dave was the blond, handsome, compactly athletic guy with the cute mustache and sideburns sitting below me in the anatomy amphitheater. He sat in the front row of every class, taking extensive notes, staring intently at the slides or the blackboard and watching the professor. I soon learned that he had a nearly photographic memory—a blessing and, eventually, a curse. He was so focused that he didn't even notice my considerable efforts at flirting.

He was driven to be the best. At everything. He studied compulsively, always seeking out extra material and opportunities to practice what he learned. Classmates turned to him for help, and he willingly and patiently tutored them. He was intense. He was complicated.

He grew up relying on sports to serve as an emotional outlet and help maintain an even keel in life. But medical school was so time-consuming that he needed exercise which he could do at odd hours and which didn't require money or other people to participate.

So, running became his thing. Starting at 5:00 a.m., before the Inland Empire heat and smog settled in, he ran on silent, isolated, dark roads through orange grove after orange grove. He contemplated the first of thousands of sunrises. The beginning of the thousands of miles he would run, the thousands of thoughts that he would cycle through.

If you passed him on the road, you would see him talking to himself, his arms pumping and hands gesticulating. His mind raced ahead of his feet. I imagined him with cartoon bubbles flying out behind his head with endless lists: the Krebs cycle, pharmaceuticals, microbes, syndromes, and pathology. The thoughts fit with running; they both went on and on. Who knows—perhaps imaginary professors sprinted alongside him, refueling him with more lists.

If you had asked him why he was running, he would have said because it calmed him and helped temper his impulsivity for the rest of the day. That was the 1970s, and researchers were just discovering the opioid neuropeptides now known as endorphins that eventually inspired the term "runner's high." He was living proof that it is an effective process. When he didn't run, he was hard to live with. When he ran, he was easy to love.

By the end of medical school, he averaged thirty-five miles per week. When possible, I rode my mint-green Bianchi racing bike beside him. It was so light, with its sew-up racing tires, that I could sling it over my shoulder and walk when his run went off-road.

As the miles sped by, he kept solving problems and making plans. He decided what to specialize in and where to do a residency. My flirting eventually paid off. It was probably on one of these runs that he decided to marry me, the classmate with long brown hair.

O-dark-thirty. Military time became the norm as he started his radiation therapy residency at the Naval Regional Medical Center San Diego. Every exam room held a person with a cancer diagnosis; each hour-long appointment confronted life and death. Their faces betrayed fear, incomprehension, and *Why me?* thoughts. Pain sat in the room with them. Dave approached each person's problem as though it was the most important one in the world, attacking their worries with the same intensity I'd seen in school.

Each treatment plan had to be exact. His obsessive-compulsive tendencies were a great attribute now. He prescribed high doses of radiation for their tumors; the margins of the radiation beam had to be meticulously tailored to treat only the abnormal tissues. Side effects are common and can be devastating. It was just the beginning of countless nights of sleep that would be interrupted with concerns about complications.

To keep things in perspective and to stay in shape, Dave started running more. By leaving the house at 4:30 a.m., he was able to run the twelve miles to work and be ready to start the day by 7:25 each morning. He rode his bike home, repeating the twenty-four-mile run-ride cycle every day.

In 1978, Dave and his brother, Mark, started running marathons. Ramping up their training to seventy miles per week, they did two or three marathons that year and were especially proud of the day they ran a 2:59 race in January, 1979.

It was in August of that year that we went on vacation with Dave's family in Germany. Six of us were riding in a borrowed VW van that fateful afternoon, our destination Hitler's getaway, the Eagle's Nest, high up in the alpine town of Berchtesgaden, when the van stopped on the tracks and couldn't be restarted. The train barreled toward us, and I fell out onto the tracks.

Dave knew there was not enough time, but he ran the twenty yards anyway. He ran the fastest run of his life. He ran knowing that either he would save me or we would die.

Dave still runs. It's not always at O-dark-thirty these days. His shirts and shorts are now high-tech fabrics, and, while not a fashion statement, they're a little more coordinated than they were so many years ago. The mustache is sprinkled with gray. He has an abnormal EKG, which, like his personality, normalizes after running.

In his compulsive fashion, he records his running mileage every day on a San Diego tide calendar. At the end of the year, he totals it up; every year, it's between 1,700 and 1,800 miles. His times are now eight-to-nine-minute miles, and there are days when he needs to slow down or walk.

We've known each other for more than eighty thousand miles.

Forty years after the accident, he says, "Every day of my life, I think of what might have been if I had had just one more second."

Every day I think, *I still can't believe he ran fast enough to save my life!*

EPILOGUE:

A Son's Perspective

....

I think I had a normal childhood. A typical day included dodging wheelchairs, dreading Mom's vegetarian hamburgers, and being forced to practice the piano. Family vacations involved argument-filled road trips, weeklong canoeing trips into the middle of nowhere, and the key question of whether to bring along an extra pair of legs. Weekends featured San Diego Padres games, chores, and backyard butt-walk races. Most exciting was driving around empty parking lots, wearing helmets and elbow pads, squealing more loudly than the tires as Mom took a new car for a spin. Pretty close to normal for me was pretty far from normal for others.

Five years before I was born, my parents were in a train accident in Germany that left my mother a triple amputee, her left arm the only appendage remaining. She learned to walk with prosthetic legs, write with her left hand, drive a car with one arm, and make dinner from a wheelchair. Despite having to give up her favorite activities of swimming and biking, she found ways to get carried, rowed, and dragged through mountains, lakes, and fields of snow and never lost sight of her professional goals in medicine. She worked hard and became an award-winning physician. By the time she had me, she was living a new normal life.

While my mother's adaptations occurred primarily in full view, my father's actions were largely behind the scenes. At the time of the accident, Mom told Dad earnestly that if he wanted to walk away from the marriage, she would understand. Without hesitation, he informed her that he hadn't married her for her arms and legs and that they'd find ways to get over hurdles. For more than thirty years, my dad has stood unwaveringly by his word and dedicated himself to enabling a disabled woman. This complex relationship seemed completely normal to me as a child and served as the basis for my lifelong education.

My dad has shown me that a person is more than her body parts, that everyone is a character worth appreciating, that more exists than what is on the surface. As a couple, my parents reveal the dedication and effort required in a genuine partnership. I have learned that what some call sacrifice is actually a combination of compassion, respect, and willingness—even eagerness—to change for someone else.

Acknowledgments

···

D onna and Jack, Mable and Albert: Dave and I will never be able to thank you enough for molding us, your children, into strong, resilient people. You taught us to never give up, work hard, and love each other unconditionally. Your commitment to each other was the example we followed. To our siblings—Mark, Albert, and Janice—and your families, thank you for supporting us and keeping our family intact.

Without the five talented and caring Austrian surgeons, this wouldn't have been a very long story; it would have ended in the Unfallkrankenhaus, Salzburg's trauma hospital. Thank you for being ready when the ambulance rolled up and for whisking me into the operating room, and thank you also to the nurses and staff who supported us in the days following the accident. Nora, Dave still calls you our "angel" nurse. You took charge on day one and stayed in our lives for the next thirty-five years. You are missed.

We're so grateful for our family friends Adrian and Johnny Johnston, who ran the show and kept our family sane in that awful first year. Thank you for being our rock. And, Adrian, thank you for being a sounding board as I wrote this book and for verifying and remembering important or missing details.

Carla and Juli, my dear college roommates, and their husbands, Roger Cox and Barry Miller, were with us in spirit from the beginning. A thousand thank-yous for getting us back into the great outdoors and for being our travel companions. And to the Cox children, Leif and Heidi, thank you for all the ways you thought up over the years to push, pull, or carry me so our families could have fabulous wilderness adventures where we didn't see other people for days at a time. Juli, you made this book-writing adventure a lot easier because you saved all our notes and letters from the very beginning. Thank you for reading and editing most of the things I've written and for being the best friend ever.

Thank you to my attending orthopedic surgeon, John Webster, who pushed me gently every day to maximize my rehabilitation. And thank you, Donna Pavlick, for being my twenty-nine-year-old counterpart in showing the doctors who said I'd never be able to walk, or that if I did, I wouldn't go very far, that they were wrong. You were the epitome of a physical therapist. Thank you to Hugh Lacey, who readily agreed to be my obstetrician and take on the complicated task of helping a triple amputee deliver a baby. Your presence on the day Tiffany was born was a gift.

Randy Mason, thank you for fabricating my first set of legs and helping Dave pull me upright for the first time in the hospital, less than two months after the accident.

Kevin Calvo, prosthetist par excellence, if I typed "thank you" a million times, it would not convey your importance in my life. Every morning when I drive my wheelchair up to my legs, I reunite the warm, breathing upper half of my body with the cold, inanimate lower half and, thanks to you, I become whole again. You and your staff at Bionics Orthotics & Pros-thetics enabled me to be an independent and productive person.

The Navy also provided support and an extended family that helped us move forward and helped me become the doctor I'd always wanted to be. Fred Sanford and John Koval, Dave's colleagues in radiation oncology, created a work environment that allowed Dave to keep up with his residency and spend time with me in physical therapy. Thank you both. Fred and his wife, Mary Jane, and John and his wife, Laura, devoted countless hours to helping us outside the hospital as well. I'll also always be grateful for the diagnostic radiology residents who treated me as one of their own while we worried our way through oral boards preparation during my recovery in the naval hospital. Thank you for putting me in a wheelchair and taking me to noon conferences and film readout sessions in the department. Those times allowed me to envision myself as a radiologist and distracted me a little more each day from thinking about how I looked and what I couldn't do. You helped me to see what I could do in the future if I just got off my butt and did the work.

Thank you to the radiology residents, faculty, and staff at the White Memorial Medical Center who worked with me as I figured out new ways to do things after returning to work. I felt your strong arms around me during the first transatlantic phone calls while we were in Salzburg, and when we returned home, you sent radiology textbooks, hoping I'd be inspired to study. I remember Drs. Sanders, Woesner, and Braun driving to San Diego with their wives to see us a few weeks after the accident. When Dave carried me into the living room, Dr. Sanders turned on a Kodak projector loaded with slides for a lecture on cardiac radiology, which he proceeded to give as if he had an audience of hundreds. You all rallied around me in your own ways to get me back to finish my residency and pass my radiology boards. My radiology career started with you.

The radiology department at the University of California, San Diego, probably deserves its own book. Thank you for taking me under your wing in an era when women were a rarity in radiology and many years before the Americans with Disabilities Act mandated that people with disabilities be offered equal opportunities in employment. John Byfield creatively got my fake feet in the door in 1981. Jack Forrest, Paul Friedman, and Dave Feigin were luminaries in pulmonary radiology, and I was honored to learn and work alongside them. I envied Jack's ability to look at a chest film and decide instantly whether it was normal or abnormal—probably the hardest decision a radiologist makes. I will never forget Dr. Lasser saying repeatedly, "Call me Elliott." It took me months to stop saying "Dr. Lasser." I will always be in debt to John A. Amberg, who, as chief resident, urged the faculty to offer me the option of completing my residency at UCSD, and to his father, John R. Amberg, who exemplified the three *a*'s—availability, affability, and ability—and whom I tried to emulate. Bob Berk, as chairman, helped me find my niche. Barbara Gosink, thank you for putting my wheelchair in your car and driving me to radiology meetings in those first few years. Lee Talner, thanks for pushing me out to my car in a wheelchair at 5:30 p.m. on March 26, 1984, so I could get home before turning around and coming back to the hospital to deliver our son, Brian, at 9:15 that night. George Leopold, I suspect you are the only department chairman who ever put his arms around a colleague and carried her up the steps of a bus so she could attend a meeting of the University of California radiology chairs. Thank you. And to Shelley Van Buren, Vivian Cohen, Beverly Esposito, and Kathy Shepherd, thank you for being my secretaries and, therefore, my legs and arms. Without you, I'd have starved. You graciously brought me a cookie and coffee for lunch every day. There are hundreds of more names that belong on these pages. If you are reading this, please mentally add your name and a big thank you from me. I was blessed to work with all of you and in this department for thirty years.

Big thanks to Lee and Adele Parmley and Scott and Terrie Purdy, friends who weren't afraid to show up when others were hesitant, friends who laughed and cried with us at the absurdity of things. You were patient and let me try things on my own yet were there when I needed help.

Although their last names are different than ours, these women are truly part of our family: Fermina Rincon, Francis Gonzalez, and Maria Trujillo. Thank you for keeping our house clean and organized so Dave and I could manage a family while working full-time. We couldn't have done it without you. And while Tiffany and Brian were young, Phyllis, Dorrie Scheider, Michelle Fiveash, Marge Chellis, and Jackie Pohaku were the extra arm and legs that I needed to run after toddlers and keep them safe. Thank you.

Darrell Heath, please don't ever die or go out of business. Thank you for taking over the MPS company from George and Butch in 1994 and turning it into the Ability Center. The adaptive devices you've installed and maintained on my cars have allowed me to work full-time, take my kids to school, watch them play water polo, and live like every other able-bodied mom.

Joye and Ernie Mason, you were not only the best-ever neighbors but also surrogate grandparents and great role models for Tiffany and Brian. Thank you.

I cannot finish this book without shout-outs to two water polo coaches: Doug Peabody, of San Diego Shores Water Polo Club and The Bishops School, Brian and Tiffany's "other dad"; and Jamey Wright, the iconic women's water polo coach at UC Davis. Thank you for instilling the dedication, teamwork, and confidence in our children that made them into strong, capable adults.

And finally, a big thank-you to my writing mentors and buddies. This all started after Tiffany emailed me the piece she created for an online writing class at UCLA. The story about her mom and dad was so gripping that I decided if she could do it, I could do it. That essay is now the prologue of this book. Likewise, Brian's writing is so compelling that I saved the personal statement from his medical school application; it is the epilogue. Thank you to Shawna Kenney and Sharon Bray in the memoir-writing program at UCLA Extension. Attending the Community of Writers at Squaw Valley gave me the validation I needed to get serious about creating this memoir. Thank you, Judy Reeves and Marnie Freedman, for introducing me to the art of memoir writing through your evening classes at UCSD and continued mentoring through San Diego Writers Ink classes. Zoe Ghahremani, thank you for telling me that I *must* write a book about our life and then inviting me to join your writing group. I tried to ignore you, but you are one unignorable person. Before attending your group, I even found the address of your house and drove by, thinking that if it was inaccessible, I'd have an excuse not to come. Anne Valadez, Penelope James, Barbara Sack, Susan McBeth, Alice Lowe: thank you for helping bring emotion to my happy-go-lucky stories. Thanks also to Elizabeth Vaughn, Jeniffer Thompson, Kat Alexander, Katie McNeel, Tracy Jones, Anique Mautner, David Reed, Janice Alper, Connie Henry, Barb Huntington, Anne Janda, and Rose Lochmann. Marilyn Woods, somehow you always pulled one more description out of me that better animated my stories. Especially big thank yous to Julie Abbott League, Pat Eiseman, Juli Miller, Alicia Amberg and my husband Dave Hodgens for reading the final version from beginning to end. The give-and-take of writing critiques was always productive and almost always fun.

Jeniffer Thompson and Kat Endries at Monkey C Media, thank you for dragging me kicking and screaming into the digital era with a beautiful web page.

To my literary agent, Lilly Ghahremani, thank you for believing this book could and would be published and for guiding me through the complexities of the publishing industry and encouraging me every step of the way. Cristen Iris, you saw this as a love story from the moment you read it. Thank you from the bottom of my heart for taking the stories I'd written and turning them into a book. And thank you to Brooke Warner, Samantha Strom, Lauren Wise, Annie Tucker, Kristin Andrews, and Julie Metz at She Writes Press, who took a manuscript and made the finished product come to life on the printed page.

About the Author

L inda K. Olson, MD, FACR, is a graduate of Loma Linda University School of Medicine 1976-A. She completed her diagnostic radiology residency at the White Memorial Medical Center in 1981 after which she joined the faculty in the Department of Radiology, University of California at San Diego. As Director of Breast Imaging at UCSD for twenty years, she provided inspiration to women with breast cancer and mentored countless medical students and residents. She is the recipient of multiple awards, including the Academic Senate Distinguished Teaching Award from UCSD in 1996, Marie Curie Award of the American Association of Women Radiologists 1991, Honored Alumna Loma Linda University School of Medicine 1994, San Diego County's 2011 Physicians of Exceptional Excellence "Top Doctors" Award, Loma Linda University School of Medicine "Women in Courage" Award 2012, and UCSD Department of Radiology Lifetime Achievement Award 2012.

Now a Professor Emeritus of Radiology at UCSD, she is committed to empowering Parkinson's patients and families to live life as fully as possible in spite of their disabilities. She has been a triple amputee since 1979 and was diagnosed with Parkinson's disease in 2015. Olson and her husband, David Hodgens, MD, raised two children, Tiffany Hodgens and Brian Hodgens, and now live in San Diego with their black lab, Sally. This is her first book.

Learn more at www.lindakolson.com.

SELECTED TITLES FROM SHE WRITES PRESS

....

She Writes Press is an independent publishing company founded to serve women writers everywhere. Visit us at www.shewritespress.com.

Rethinking Possible: A Memoir of Resilience by Rebecca Faye Smith Galli. $16.95, 978-1-63152-220-8. After her brother's devastatingly young death tears her world apart, Becky Galli embarks upon a quest to recreate the sense of family she's lost—and learns about healing and the transformational power of love over loss along the way.

A Leg to Stand On: An Amputee's Walk into Motherhood by Colleen Haggerty. $16.95, 978-1-63152-923-8. Haggerty's candid story of how she overcame the pain of losing a leg at seventeen— and of terminating two pregnancies as a young woman—and went on to become a mother, despite her fears.

Body 2.0: Finding My Edge Through Loss and Mastectomy by Krista Hammerbacher Haapala. An authentic, inspiring guide to reframing adversity that provides a new perspective on preventative mastectomy, told through the lens of the author's personal experience.

Off the Rails: One Family's Journey Through Teen Addiction by Susan Burrowes. $16.95, 978-1-63152-467-7. An inspiring story of family love, determination, and the last-resort intervention that helped one troubled young woman find sobriety after a terrifying and harrowing journey.

A Different Kind of Same: A Memoir by Kelley Clink. $16.95, 978-1-63152-999-3. Several years before Kelley Clink's brother hanged himself, she attempted suicide by overdose. In the aftermath of his death, she traces the evolution of both their illnesses, and wonders: If he couldn't make it, what hope is there for her?

Hug Everyone You Know: A Year of Community, Courage, and Cancer by Antoinette Truglio Martin. $16.95, 978-1-63152-262-8. Cancer is scary enough for the brave, but for a wimp like Antoinette Martin, it was downright terrifying. With the help of her community, however, Martin slowly found the courage within herself to face cancer—and to do so with perseverance and humor.